40 DAYS TO
BETTER LIVING
DEPRESSION

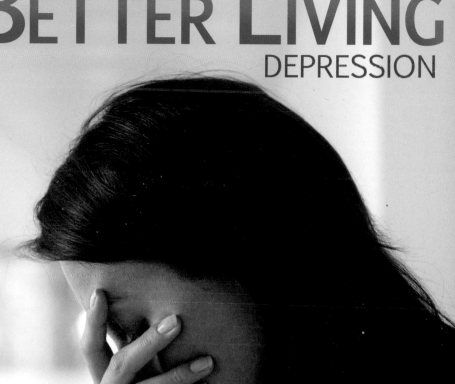

BARBOUR
PUBLISHING

Published by Barbour Publishing, Inc., P.O. Box 719, Uhrichsville, Ohio 44683, www.barbourbooks.com

Our mission is to publish and distribute inspirational products offering exceptional value and biblical encouragement to the masses.

 Member of the
Evangelical Christian
Publishers Association

Printed in the United States of America.

CONTENTS

Welcome, from Dr. Scott Morris,
Founder of the Church Health Center

Week 1: Liz's Story

Starting Out / First Steps / Beginning the Journey / Acknowledging
Our Feelings / One Day at a Time / Reaching Out / Celebration!

Week 2: Nadia's Story

Finding Balance / Letting Go / Isolation / Patience /
Managing Our Feelings / Hope / Knowing Joy

Week 3: Greg's Story

Feeling Rested / Forms of Rest / Making Space / Being Intentional /
Asking for Help / Sustaining Rest / Halfway There

Week 4: Michael's Story

The Process / Experiencing Setbacks / Our Attitude / Physical
Depression / Reviving Our Spirit / Joy / Our Whole Self

Week 5: Ada's Story

A New People / Letting Go / Reuniting with Ourselves / The Slow
Transformation / Hope and Energy / A Fresh Start / The Light Ahead

Week 6: Dawn's Story

Your Story / Seeing Ourselves / Next Steps / Encouragement / Forty
Days! / Review / Looking Ahead

Recommended Reading and Resources.

Welcome,
From Dr. Scott Morris,
Founder of the Church Health Center

I first came to Memphis in 1986. I had no personal ties to Memphis and did not know anyone here. Having completed theological and medical education, I was determined to begin a health care ministry for the working poor. The next year, the doors of the Church Health Center opened with one doctor—me—and one nurse. We saw 12 patients the first day. Today we handle about 36,000 patient visits each year and 120,000 visits to our wellness facility. A staff of 250 people share a ministry of healing and wellness, and hundreds more volunteer time and services.

So what sets us apart from other community clinics around the country?

The Church Health Center is fundamentally about the church. We care for our patients without relying on government funds, because God calls the church to healing work. Jesus' life was about healing the whole person—body and spirit—and the church is Jesus in the world. His message is our message. His ministry is our ministry. Local congregations embrace this calling and help make our work possible.

More than two decades of caring for the working uninsured makes one thing plain: health care needs to change. In the years that the

> Jesus' life was about healing the whole person— body and spirit. . .

Church Health Center has cared for people in Memphis, we have seen that two-thirds of our patients seek treatment for illness that healthier living can prevent or control. We realized that if we want to make a lasting difference in our patients' lives, the most effective strategy is to encourage overall wellness in body and spirit. At a fundamental level, we must transform what the words *well* and *health* mean in the minds of most people.

To do that, we developed the Model for Healthy Living. Living healthy lives doesn't just mean that you see the doctor regularly. Rather, healthy living means that all aspects of your life are in balance. Your faith, work, nutrition, movement, family and friends, emotions, and medical health all contribute to a life filled with more joy, more love, and more connection with God.

How to Use This Book

This book provides opportunities to improve your health in whatever way you need to for your optimal wellness. For the next forty days, we invite you to be inspired by the real-life people whose lives have been changed by the Church Health Center. Each day offers us a new chance to improve our health, so each day we will give you helpful ways that you can make your life healthier.

Some days you may choose to focus on just one or two of our "tips": Faith Life, Medical, Movement, Work, Emotional, Family and Friends, or Nutrition. Some days you may want to try all of them. The important thing is to remember that God calls us to an abundant life, and we can always make changes to strive for our optimal wellness.

Forty days and numerous ways to live a healthy life—come and join us on the journey!

Five years ago, Liz came to the Church Heath Center feeling like she needed a change. She

set a goal to lose ten pounds and she found the Wellness classes helpful and enjoyed the walking track.

But after she had been here for about a year, she experienced some major setbacks that didn't have much to do with her exercise or nutrition. She lost her job and had a tough time finding another one, and her long-term relationship ended. Then, when her father lost a long-fought battle to cancer, Liz began to feel depressed. She started to lose interest in exercising, eating well, and wellness in general. She gained back the weight she had lost and ate poorly and sporadically. Even her favorite meals from the Wellness Kitchen didn't seem to taste right anymore.

As her overall health started to deteriorate, her doctor recommended that she see a counselor. "I didn't think of myself as depressed, but I just felt so down. It was a struggle to motivate myself to do anything," she says. Her counselor recommended talk therapy and encouraged her to get back on her wellness regimen.

"I didn't really feel like working out at first, but the encouragement from another person really helped." Liz went back to her cooking class, started working out on a regular basis, and saw a counselor once a month. Eventually, she started to feel more "normal" again. "I still have good days and bad days, but even on bad days, I feel like it's easier to manage when I stick with my classes and exercise."

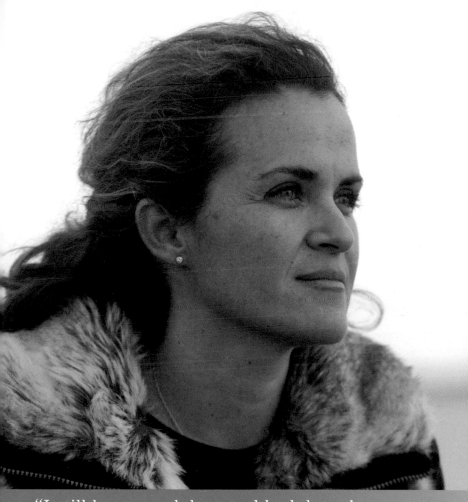

"I still have good days and bad days, but even on bad days, I feel like it's easier to manage when I stick with my classes and exercise."

Depression

Morning Reflection

Congratulations! Today you are taking the first step on a journey toward wellness and managing your depression. On this six-week journey, we will work to make lifestyle changes that will help you to manage depression and live a wellness-oriented life. But every journey has a beginning—a first day or a first step. These first days may feel difficult and overwhelming, but we can find comfort in knowing that God walks all of our steps with us, including the difficult ones.

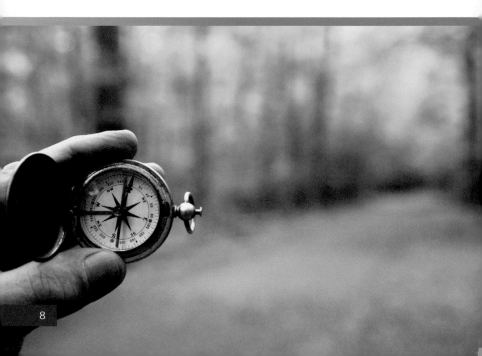

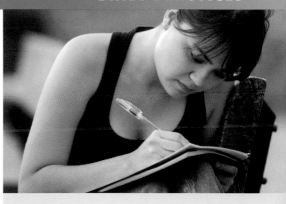

»Faith Life

Today, write a couple of sentences about what role faith plays in your life. Do you belong to a church? Do you spend time reading the Bible? Do you pray? This will help you gauge where you go as you continue on this journey.

No, No,
Yes - through
out the day

> { "I didn't really feel like working out at first, but the encouragement from another person really helped." }

»Medical

As we begin this journey, it is important to know where we stand. Make a list of any medical conditions for which you are currently being treated and/or monitored.

1 *Bp*
2 *Moodswings*
3

»Movement

Often, depression has physical symptoms, such as muscular aches and pains. Today, try to do some mild stretching. Roll your neck. Stretch out your shoulders. Bend down and try to touch your toes. How does it feel to let your body move?

9

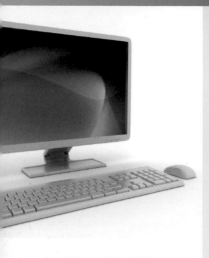

»Work

Do you spend a lot of time at work staring at a computer screen or performing repetitive actions? Today, keep a log of how much time you spend doing the same thing.

»Emotional

Today, set aside a place to keep a journal. Use a notebook, the computer, this book, or whatever works for you. In the weeks to come, it will be very helpful to have one place for journaling exercises.

»Family and Friends

Having a support system is very important in managing depression. Today, make a list of family and friends or other people who will be there to support you on this journey.

»Nutrition

Today when you eat, try to taste everything that you consume. We can often find ourselves swallowing food without really tasting it. As we learn to taste, we can learn to eat healthier.

Evening Wrap-up

We all have beginnings, and we all have first steps. The first days of any journey can be intimidating, because we are not always certain what lies ahead on the journey. But even God experienced the beginning of a journey: "The earth was formless and empty." We might feel that our futures are formless and empty at the beginning of a journey, especially when it is a path to change our lives. But now, in the beginning, we can remember that God made all of creation from a formless and empty void. Surely, God will walk with us on this journey.

In the beginning God created the heavens and the earth. Now the earth was formless and empty, darkness was over the surface of the deep, and the Spirit of God was hovering over the waters.

Genesis 1:1–2

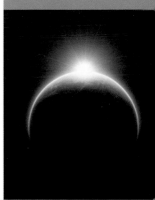

God of new beginnings, grant me courage and serenity as I embark on this journey toward wellness. Help me to shape my life to be healthier and happier. In Your holy name, Amen.

Morning Reflection

Any time we decide to make a change in course, the transition can be difficult. Making those changes can be even more difficult when we feel like we don't have the physical and emotional energy necessary to make those changes. Depression can really rob us of that energy and can make wellness seem like an impossible goal. Today, we will focus on how we can move forward even when it seems like we lack the energy to do so.

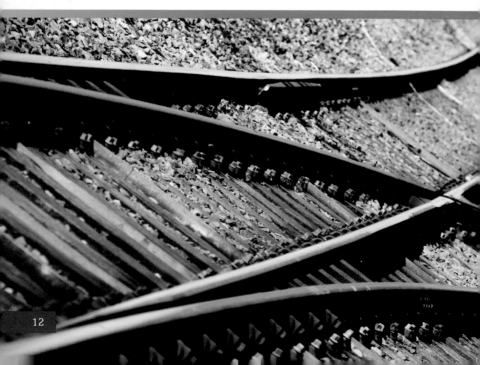

»Faith Life

Meditation can be a very valuable practice in faith life and in managing depression. Today, spend three minutes sitting quietly and focusing on your breathing. Try to quiet your inner voices as much as you are able.

{ Today, we will focus on how we can move forward even when it seems like we lack the energy to do so. }

»Medical

Make a list of your prescribed medications today. Include where they are to be stored (refrigerator, medicine cabinet) and how often you take them. Hang the list on your refrigerator, or put it in another easy-to-find location.

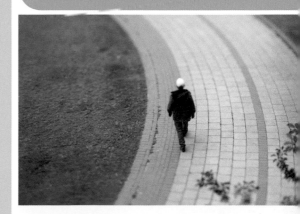

»Movement

Today, go for a short walk. Walk around your neighborhood, around a park, around your office—wherever is most comfortable and convenient for you. Try to get your heart rate up a bit, and make sure that you drink plenty of water.

» Work

What is your work? Remember that what we call "work" includes your job, your volunteer work, raising children, etc. Today spend five minutes writing about your work.

» Emotional

Today, in your journal, take an "emotional inventory." Try to write down as many words as possible that describe how you are feeling. *Tired? Frustrated? Anxious? Eager?* Write for at least five minutes.

» Family and Friends

Today, go for a short walk with a friend or a family member. Focus on feeling your body move as well as enjoying the company. Having a partner on the journey can be very helpful!

» Nutrition

Do you have a standard list for the grocery store? Make a list of things that you normally buy when you shop. In the days and weeks to come, change your grocery list based on the dietary suggestions made.

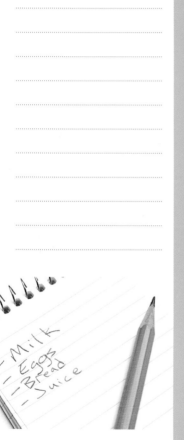

Evening Wrap-up

Changing course can truly feel

like misery. It can leave us feeling lost, even on the best of days when we are trying to manage and deal with depression, changing course can appear large and daunting on the horizon. But the prophet Micah tells us that change includes both sadness and hope. "As for me, I watch in hope for the LORD. . . . God will hear me." Today, we can remember that God hears us, even in the midst of misery and desolation.

What misery is mine! I am like one who gathers summer fruit at the gleaning of the vineyard; there is no cluster of grapes to eat, none of the early figs that I crave. The faithful have been swept from the land; not one upright person remains. . . . But as for me, I watch in hope for the LORD, I wait for God my Savior; my God will hear me.

MICAH 7:1–2, 7

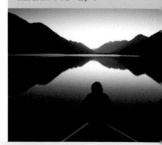

God of hope, give me the voice to reach out to You even as I feel hopeless. Give me the strength to find hope in You. Thank You for hearing me. In Your holy name, Amen.

Morning Reflection

Liz's wellness journey began a year before she became depressed. While we can say that each day is a new beginning (and it is!), there are some journeys that require many days—or even weeks—to really begin in earnest. The journey to wellness in our body and spirit is one of those journeys. Today, on Day Three, it is important to remember that we are still in the early days. We are beginning changes that will last a lifetime. But these changes take time and require that we be patient and gracious with ourselves.

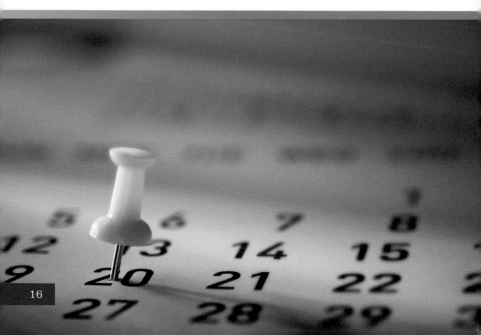

» Faith Life

Do you pray before meals? If you do not, try it today. Sometimes it helps to find even the smallest moment to remember that God is at work in your life. Simply take a moment to be thankful before you start eating.

» Medical

Depression can be triggered by a larger medical issue. When was your last physical from a medical doctor? If it has been more than a year, call your doctor and make an appointment today.

» Movement

Today, after your shower, when your muscles are warm, do some light stretching. If any stretches hurt, stop doing them. You should feel only some mild discomfort when stretching.

» Work

What do you enjoy about your work? What do you dislike? What do you find stressful about your work? Today, take five minutes and write about your likes and dislikes about your work.

» Emotional

Depression can be triggered by stress, so today, spend five minutes practicing deep breathing. Take a deep breath in through your nose and slowly let it out through your mouth. This is a wonderful exercise for moments when you begin to feel overwhelmed.

» Family and Friends

When was the last time you had a family dinner? Family dinners can be a wonderful way to spend time laughing and talking with people you love. They are also a great time to try out new recipes. Today, think of a time when you had an enjoyable dinner with some family and friends. What made that meal special?

» Nutrition

Your nutrition can affect your emotional health. Eating a healthy and diverse diet can help you to feel energized and healthy. Today, write down a simple nutritional goal to focus on for the next few weeks.

But now in Christ Jesus you who once were far away have been brought near by the blood of Christ. For he himself is our peace. . . . Consequently, you are no longer foreigners and strangers, but fellow citizens with God's people and also members of his household. . . . And in him you too are being built together to become a dwelling in which God lives by his Spirit.

EPHESIANS 2:13–14, 19, 22

Evening Wrap-up

Depression is a very difficult emotional state, not just because it affects our emotional stability, but also because it skews our entire perception of reality. When we are "in" our depression, it can feel nearly impossible to see the value within ourselves. But in his letter to the Ephesians, Paul reminds us that God is building us to become a dwelling for God's Spirit. Our reality is that God dwells with us and in us.

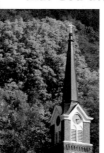

God within us, help me to be gracious with myself, and give me the perspective to see the value that You see in me. In Your holy name, Amen.

Morning Reflection

When we are managing depression, feelings of hopelessness and exhaustion often go together. But the journey to wellness is about recognizing that, even in the midst of those feelings, we have the resources at our disposal to get help and to begin again. Liz was able to get help only after she recognized that she was "feeling down." One of the first steps on the journey is to learn to acknowledge those feelings and recognize that those feelings are not the end of the story.

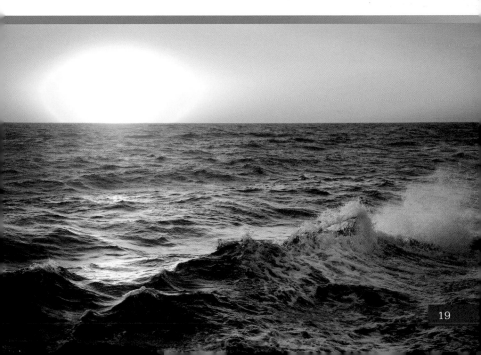

»Medical

Have you talked to your doctor about your emotional state? Many of us do not think of discussing our emotions with a physician, but it can be important information for your doctor when thinking about your overall health.

»Movement

Go for a walk today, walking as far as you can go without exhausting yourself. How far would you like to be able to walk by the end of this journey?

»Work

What do you usually do on your breaks? Do you drink coffee? Eat a snack? Today, try going for a short walk (outside if possible). Getting a little bit of exercise can lift your mood and give you a much-needed pick-me-up.

»Faith Life

How would you like to see your faith life change over the next several weeks? Today, take five minutes and write three goals for your faith life while you are on this journey.

{ One of the first steps on the journey is to learn to acknowledge those feelings and recognize that those feelings are not the end of the story. }

»Emotional

Each day has its own emotional land-scape—ups and downs. Today, write in your journal about an emotional high point as well as an emotional low point. What were the events that happened immediately before and after both of these points?

»Family and Friends

Are you embarking on this journey on your own or with a friend or some family members? Being on the journey with another person can give you an instant support group as you progress. Today, think of a friend or family member who might help you on this journey.

»Nutrition

Our emotional stability can be affected by our stomachs. Skipping meals or eating overly sugary foods can result in emotional highs followed by a severe crash. Today, try to focus on eating healthy, nutrient-dense snacks (such as nuts, fruit, or a cup of yogurt) when you feel hungry. Do not skip meals!

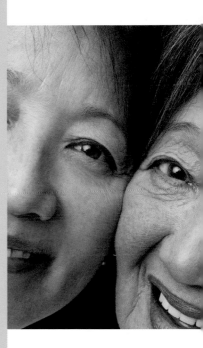

"If only my anguish could be weighed and all my misery be placed on the scales! It would surely outweigh the sand of the seas—no wonder my words have been impetuous. The arrows of the Almighty are in me, my spirit drinks in their poison; God's terrors are marshaled against me."

JOB 6:2–4

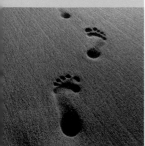

Evening Wrap-up

Job's story is one of the most profound expressions of despair and hopelessness available to us. He wails that his misery "would surely outweigh the sand of the seas." He even goes so far as to ask God for a quick death. He wants to die! But in the midst of that misery, God does not turn a deaf ear to Job. God does not turn a deaf ear to us, even when we are in the midst of despair and hopelessness. God is with us and hears our cries.

Loving and Eternal God, help me today to acknowledge my feelings and trust that You hear me, even when I cannot see the hope that You offer me. In Your holy name, Amen.

Morning Reflection

This morning marks yet another beginning, another new start, another day on the journey. But at this point, we may start to look to the weeks ahead and feel that we will never achieve the level of wellness that we desire. We can begin to feel overwhelmed, which can lead to feeling stuck. Even the smallest steps forward can become difficult. Today, we will focus on how to take the journey one day at a time.

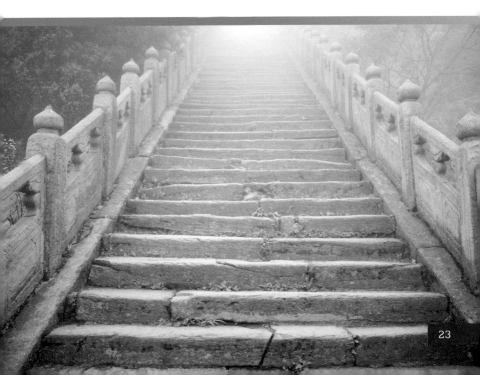

» Faith Life

Most of us have had both significant and minor setbacks in faith at some point in our lives. Think of a time when you experienced a setback in your faith life and how you managed to move forward.

» Medical

Do you smoke? If so, now is the time to quit. Depression is significantly more difficult to manage while smoking on a regular basis. Talk with your medical caregiver about safe and effective ways that you can kick the habit.

» Movement

Today spend five minutes getting your heart rate up—try doing jumping jacks or walking up a flight of stairs. Getting even a little bit of exercise can help lift your mood.

» Work

How do setbacks affect your work? Do you become less engaged in work? Or do you throw yourself into work? Today, think of something you can keep at work that can help you alleviate stress. Maybe it's a plant or a postcard, a stress ball or a mini basketball hoop. Find one thing you can keep close by to reduce stress.

» Emotional

Have you seen a therapist or counselor? If you have not, try to make an appointment today. One-on-one counseling can help with managing even mild and temporary depression.

» Family and Friends

Sometimes we can feel that our family and friends have particular expectations of us, and that can add to stress that we are already feeling. Today, talk to a friend or family member about your journey and what your expectations are.

» Nutrition

What kind of food do you like to eat? Take five minutes and make a list of your favorite foods. Are they healthy foods? Comfort foods? As this journey progresses, you may be able to modify your favorite foods to healthier versions.

Evening Wrap-up

We are still in the first days of our journey toward wellness, and when we look forward, we might feel overwhelmed with all we want to accomplish in the next six weeks. But today we can remember that God is walking this journey with us. God "speaks and summons the earth from the rising of the sun to where it sets." God is in the rising and the setting of the sun, and God loves us and walks this journey with us.

The Mighty One, God, the LORD, speaks and summons the earth from the rising of the sun to where it sets. From Zion, perfect in beauty, God shines forth. Our God comes and will not be silent. . . . And the heavens proclaim his righteousness, for he is a God of justice.

PSALM 50:1–3, 6

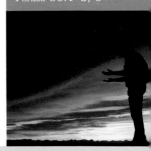

Gracious Lord, today, make me thankful for Your presence with me. Keep me mindful, even on my darkest days, that You are on this journey with me. Amen.

Morning Reflection

We have nearly reached the end of the first week! It may feel like time flies, or it may feel like it took all the effort in the world just to get to this point. Whatever our particular experience, the important thing is that we have gotten here. But as we move forward, we must realize that this journey is not one that we can walk alone. Today, we will focus on ways to reach out on our journey toward wellness.

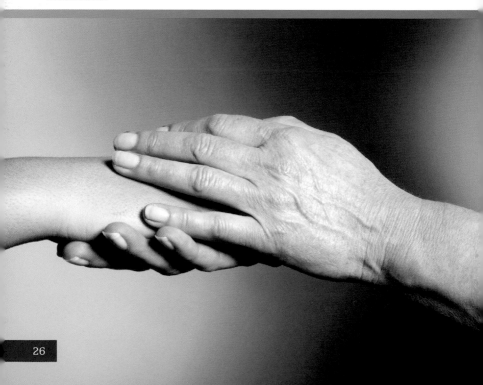

»Faith Life

On your journey, it is important to have a community of support, which can come from a faith community. Try joining a Sunday school class or a Bible study at your church to reach out to a community.

{ Today, we will focus on ways to reach out on our journey toward wellness. }

»Medical

Do you know when to seek help immediately? If you are having any thoughts of hurting yourself or others, get professional help immediately. Call your doctor, call 911, or call a national suicide hotline: 1-800-SUICIDE or 1-800-273-TALK.

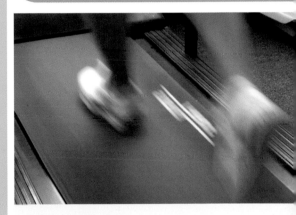

»Movement

A great way to be a part of a community and to get regular exercise is to join a nonprofit gym. They often have flexible rates to account for income differences, and they offer classes and trainers at discounted rates. Today, try to find a gym like this in your community and aks how you can join or support their efforts.

» Work

Make sure that you are well hydrated throughout the day, even if you are just sitting for most of the day. When you stay hydrated, your body works more efficiently and you will have more energy and will feel better.

» Emotional

If you start to feel overwhelmed today, sit down, close your eyes, and breathe deeply. Keep your breathing slow and even for a full minute. This will help your body to relax.

» Family and Friends

What kind of support do you need from your family and friends? Take a few minutes to identify the kind of support that would be most helpful from your personal relationships, and then talk to a friend or family member about it.

» Nutrition

One of the first steps in good nutrition is to begin reading labels on the food that you buy and eat. Go to your pantry and read the labels on ten items, taking note of sodium content. Note which foods have the highest sodium.

Evening Wrap-up

Managing depression feels like a

very lonely journey at times. After all, when we are in the midst of depression, we have a tendency to isolate ourselves. This passage from Lamentations expresses how isolating depression can be: "There is no one to comfort me." But we know that God walks the journey with us, and God can help us to reach out when we need to.

"This is why I weep and my eyes overflow with tears. No one is near to comfort me, no one to restore my spirit. . . . See, LORD, how distressed I am! I am in torment within, and in my heart I am disturbed, for I have been most rebellious. . . . People have heard my groaning, but there is no one to comfort me."

LAMENTATIONS 1:16, 20–21

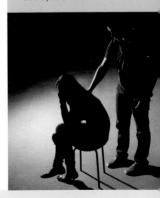

God in our midst, help me to reach out when I feel like there is no one to comfort me. Remind me that You are my comfort and my strength. Amen.

Morning Reflection

Congratulations! We have made it through the first week! Now that we are a week into our journey, we can celebrate taking those first steps toward wellness and managing depression. And as we celebrate, we can look forward to the next steps on the journey in the weeks to come.

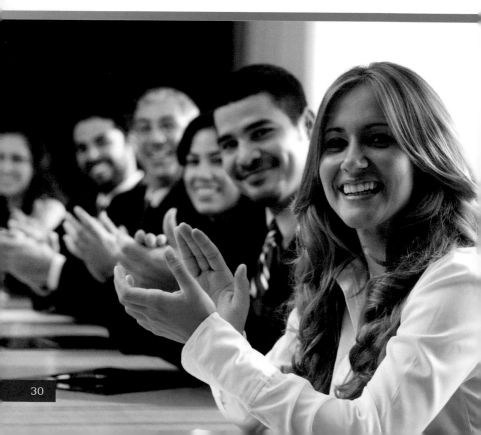

»Faith Life

Faith is an important part of wellness, but wellness is also important to faith. Keep in mind that Jesus entered this world as a person with a body. Go for a walk today, and pray as you walk for God to be present in your body as well as your spirit.

{
Congratulations!
We have reached
the end of the
first week.
}

»Medical

Do you take any herbal/mineral supplements? There are some herbal supplements that can help with managing depression, but be sure to check with your health care provider before starting any of them, as they can interact with medications in unexpected ways sometimes.

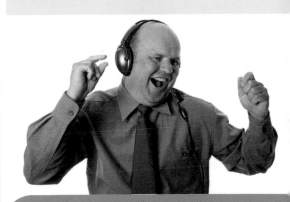

»Movement

Today, turn on some music and dance around for ten minutes. Try to let your inhibitions go and really let your body move. You may feel silly, and if you do, go ahead and laugh at yourself.

»Work

Take some small (two-to-five-pound) hand weights to work to keep at your desk. If you have a minute or two, do a few sets of simple bicep curls to work your upper body a bit.

»Emotional

Take five minutes and write in your journal about how it feels to have completed an entire week. Do you feel accomplished? Scared of what is next? Excited?

»Family and Friends

Have a small celebration with your family or some friends for getting through your first week. Do something that you enjoy doing with your family.

»Nutrition

Make a grocery list that looks forward. Include plenty of whole grains, fresh (or frozen) vegetables and fruits, and limit the prepared and processed foods. These foods tend to have more sugar and salt than other fresh foods.

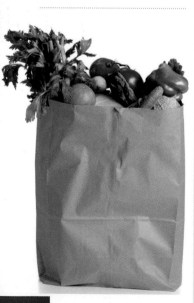

Evening Wrap-up

At the end of this first week, we celebrate the completion of our first milestone and move on to the next steps of the journey. At the end of this week, we celebrate the steps behind us as well as the steps ahead of us. And we can celebrate that God walks this journey with each of us. After all, this is the Lord who "formed you in the womb." This is the God who has made all things, and this God walks the journey with us—every step of the way.

"This is what the LORD says—your Redeemer, who formed you in the womb: I am the LORD, the Maker of all things, who stretches out the heavens, who spreads out the earth by myself."

ISAIAH 44:24

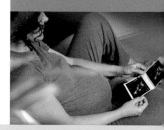

Joyous God, thank You for walking this journey with me. I know that You formed me in the womb and that You know me. Give me the strength to continue the journey from here. In Your holy name, Amen.

Nadia had felt "off" for years. She had never been horribly depressed, but always had a low-level, persistent feeling that something was wrong. She tried to make changes in her life to make things better. She got a dog, thinking that a companion would be helpful. She got rid of the TV so she wouldn't spend so much time on the couch. She even left her job and moved to another one closer to home, thinking that a shorter commute would make things a little easier. But none of these external things seemed to do the trick.

One day she began to look back over her journals from childhood. Nadia was struck at how it seemed that she had been suffering from depression for longer than she thought—even since she was a child! She began to realize that her depression wasn't something that was connected to the TV or her job. It was something ongoing and persistent in her life, and she would have to make changes in herself, not just in her environment, to deal with the depression.

She began coming to the Church Health Center, exercising, seeing a counselor, and watching her diet. Those small changes made a difference in her overall mood. She realized that the small changes, like walking and watching her diet, made more of a difference than the bigger changes, like moving! Nadia now enjoys the progress she has made at the Church Health Center, and she and her dog enjoy walking together.

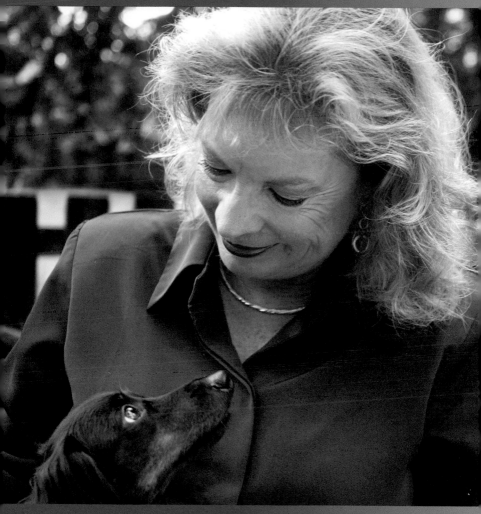

She began to realize that her depression wasn't something that was connected to the TV or her job.

Morning Reflection

Depression almost never has a simple one-stop solution—whether it's medication, therapy, getting rid of a television, or changing your diet. Managing depression, instead, means learning where your own personal balance is. Nadia had to find her own balance, making changes to her environment and lifestyle and finding outside help in the form of a counselor. We each need to find our own balance. In fact, the journey toward wellness is all about finding the balance that works for each of us to live and thrive.

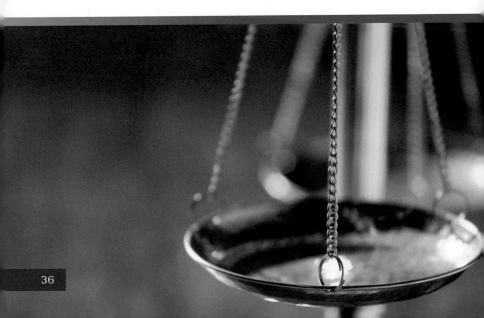

Evening Wrap-up

Depression can often make us feel off-kilter and out of balance, and so we must find our balance in the midst of depression. This verse from Ecclesiastes reminds us that God created this world with a natural balance, and so finding our own balance in the midst of God's creation is simply a part of living in this world.

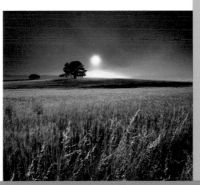

There is a time for everything, and a season for every activity under the heavens: a time to be born and a time to die, a time to plant and a time to uproot . . . a time to weep and a time to laugh, a time to mourn and a time to dance. . .a time to be silent and a time to speak, a time to love and a time to hate.

ECCLESIASTES 3:1–2, 4, 7–8

Loving God, help me to find balance on my journey to wellness. Give me the wisdom to see the balance in Your creation. In Your holy name, Amen.

Morning Reflection

When we are trying to find balance, sometimes we have to let go of our desire to control everything around us. Finding balance can be realizing where we have control and where we do not. When we try to control the things that are not ours to control, we can easily find ourselves overwhelmed and immobilized, unable to move forward. So today, we will focus on finding balance by letting go of those things over which we have no control.

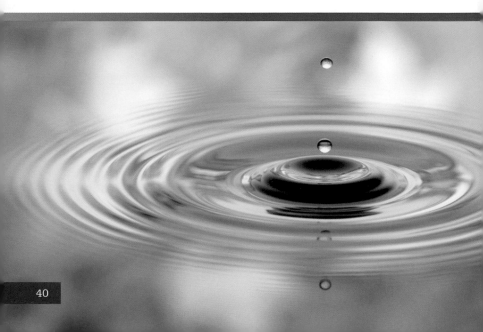

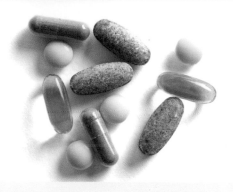

»Faith Life

Most of us have heard the phrase, "Let go and let God." What does that mean for you? Today, write a prayer in your journal for letting go.

»Medical

Make sure that you add any herbal supplements to your list of medications. If you ever have an emergency, it is important for your caregivers to know what, exactly, you are taking.

»Movement

A healthy exercise regimen consists of building our aerobic strength, muscular strength and endurance, and flexibility. Today, do three sets of ten wall push-ups to start building your upper-body strength.

{ So today, we will focus on finding balance by letting go of those things over which we have no control. }

» Work

There are some aspects of your work that you can control. Today, make a list of five workplace habits that you would like to change and that you have the power to change.

» Emotional

Recognizing when we can or cannot control a situation can help us maintain our emotional stability when we get into stressful situations. Today, write about one stressor in your life that you can control and one that you cannot.

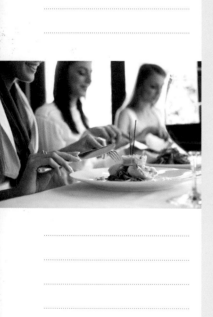

» Family and Friends

Spending time with family and friends can be a great way to relax and let go of the day. Today, gather with some friends or family to have a good meal at the end of the day.

» Nutrition

Instead of a cooked appetizer, try putting out some sliced-up fruits and vegetables. Try serving hummus or baba ganoush (roasted eggplant dip) rather than a cream- or mayonnaise-based dipping sauce (like French onion or ranch dressing).

Evening Wrap-up

While it can be very difficult to let go of the control that many of us want to have, it is important to our overall wellness that we know when to let go. Sometimes that means simply recognizing that we do not have the control we thought we had. Other times it means relying on other people or God. Jesus says, "Believe in God; trust also in me." When we trust, we let go a little and we relax a bit, and we take one more step toward wellness and health.

"Do not let your hearts be troubled. You believe in God; believe also in me. My Father's house has many rooms; if that were not so, would I have told you that I am going there to prepare a place for you?"

JOHN 14:1–2

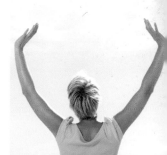

God of peace, grant me the strength and the wisdom to recognize the difference between the things I can control and the things I can't, and help me to find peace in the balance. In Your holy name, Amen.

Morning Reflection

Last week, we discussed some ways that depression can be very isolating. While we are in the midst of our depression, we might lack motivation to reach out, or we might feel like no one cares enough to respond to us. Regardless of the reason for our isolation, the truth is that on the journey toward wellness, we must find ways to get out of the pattern of isolation. We must find ways to reach out.

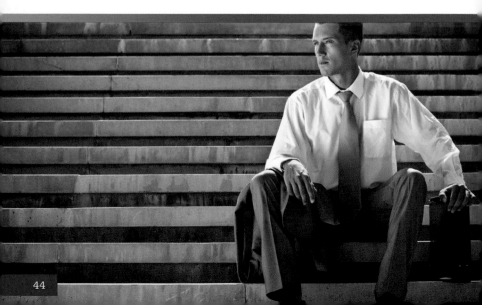

» Faith Life

Are you part of a faith community? Your church can be a wonderful resource for finding ways to reach out. If you are having trouble reaching out, try speaking with a clergy member about ways that you can get involved in the community.

» Medical

Do you know your family history? If your parents/grandparents/aunts/uncles have/had an illness, it can be relevant to your own health. Heart disease, diabetes, and cancers are particularly important to know. Along with your list of medications, include a family history of major medical problems.

» Movement

We all like to relax by watching television or reading a book. But that must be balanced by some kind of movement. Today, if you spend time watching television, try doing some bicep curls with hand weights, or do several sets of squats.

» Work

Do you work in an office where someone is always bringing in treats—birthday cake, donuts, or bagels? Balance out some of these unhealthy snacks by bringing in a fruit plate to share. Maybe you'll inspire some healthier snacks next time!

» Emotional

Today, in your journal, take an emotional inventory of yourself. How are you feeling today? Compare it to your emotional inventory from last week. What is different? What is similar?

» Family and Friends

Do you have a loved one who would be willing to check in on you once a week? Today, ask a friend or a family member to have tea (or coffee, or go for a walk) with you once a week.

» Nutrition

Today, with a friend or family member, cook a meal that has many different colors in it. Try a stir-fry with mixed vegetables, such as asparagus, red and yellow peppers, and mushrooms. Include a whole grain such as brown rice or quinoa.

We were therefore buried with him through baptism into death in order that, just as Christ was raised from the dead through the glory of the Father, we too may live a new life. For if we have been united with him in a death like his, we will certainly also be united with him in a resurrection like his.

ROMANS 6:4–5

Evening Wrap-up

Making the decision to reach out in the midst of depression can be very difficult. But on the journey toward wellness, it is important that we learn, even in small ways, to find support when we need it. As we struggle to reach out, we find help knowing that there is One who has already reached out to us. Paul reminds us in his letter to the Romans that even in the midst of our struggles, Christ reaches out to us.

God of creation, thank You for reaching out to me. Help me to reach out to others. In Your holy name, Amen.

Morning Reflection

In some ways, the journey toward wellness is never complete, and it is certainly not completed overnight. We take action when we can, but a great deal of the journey includes waiting and being patient. After all, we won't necessarily feel the changes immediately, and even when we do, they might be so gradual that it feels like we are making no progress at all. Those are the times when we need to step back and realize that with patience and perseverance, we can continue on the journey.

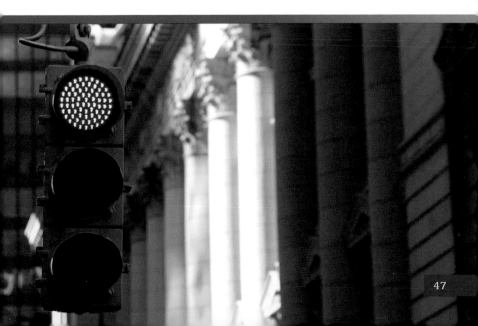

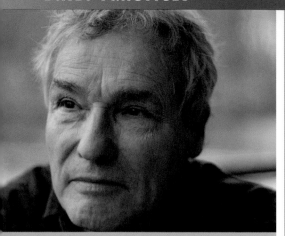

»Faith Life

Today, spend ten minutes in quiet meditation. Try to focus on finding a quiet space within yourself. Reflect on your faith journey thus far and how God has been present with you.

»Medical

Keep in mind that quick fixes in medicine are generally not a good long-term solution. The next time you have a doctor's appointment, talk to your care provider about your long-term health goals.

»Movement

To build endurance, you need to occasionally push your limits. Today, do as many jumping jacks as you can, take a one-minute break, and then do it again. Try that three times throughout the day.

{ Try to focus on finding a quiet space within yourself. }

»Work

We often focus on the negative effects of work, but working—being active and positively engaged—is an important component of wellness. Today, try to focus on the positive engagement in your work, whether you work in an office or at home.

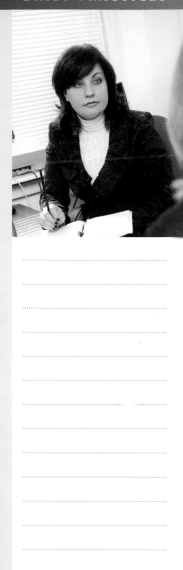

»Emotional

Today, take ten minutes and write in your journal about what waiting means to you. Do you find it difficult to wait? What are the things that you are waiting for now?

»Family and Friends

Your family and friends can make waiting feel more bearable. Today, try going for a walk with a loved one. Try to enjoy the company and the movement.

»Nutrition

Be very cautious with "fad diets" that promise quick and extreme results (such as losing thirty pounds in a month or washboard abs in just three weeks). Such diets are often unbalanced and temporary. You will be better off with long-term lifestyle changes, even though they won't "work" as rapidly.

We wait in hope for the Lord; he is our help and our shield. In him our hearts rejoice, for we trust in his holy name. May your unfailing love be with us, Lord, even as we put our hope in you.

Psalm 33:20–22

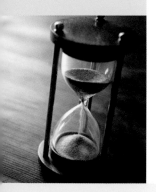

Evening Wrap-up

In our culture of fast food, overnight

delivery, and other types of instant gratification, it can be frustrating and demoralizing to keep on day after day without feeling results. In particular, when struggling with depression, we just want to feel better—yesterday! But the psalmist offers us some words of wisdom. We wait in hope. We are not guaranteed instant results, but we are hopeful. On the journey toward wellness we can persevere in hope, even on the days when we cannot feel the difference between today and two weeks ago.

Merciful Lord, thank You for walking this journey with me. Today, grant me patience on this journey toward wellness. In Your holy name, Amen.

Morning Reflection

There is a perception that managing depression is only a matter of putting on a happy face. We tell ourselves that if we were just "strong enough" we would not feel the way that we are feeling. But the truth is, managing depression is something other than "getting happy." Managing depression is about learning to accept the feelings that we have without those feelings getting the final word. It is about balancing our strengths with our weaknesses and acknowledging the struggle.

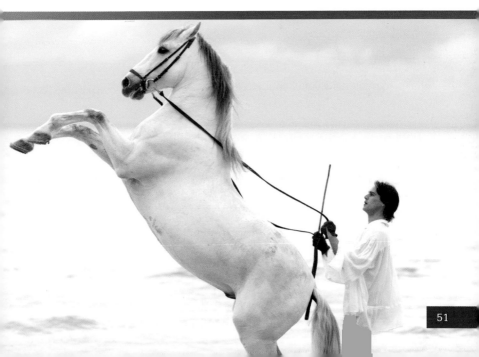

» Faith Life

Faith is a very important part of balancing your strength and weakness.
Today, take five minutes and write about how embracing your vulnerability might
help you on your faith journey.

» Medical

Our medical model is often based on what we must *do*. Exercise, eat right, and
take the right medications. But rest is just as important. Sleep gives your body the
energy to function healthily. Today, try to give yourself some rest.

» Movement

Sometimes when we are bored, our default destination is the refrigerator. We
eat when we feel bored or even tired. Today, if you feel bored, instead of eating, go
for a walk or do some jumping jacks. Try moving instead of eating.

» Work

Do you notice a time of day when you get hungry? Do you crave a specific
food when you take your break? This may be habitual eating. Today, when you feel
hungry at work, drink some water, or snack on some carrot sticks instead of head-
ing for the vending machines.

» Emotional

Write in your journal a list of your strengths and your weaknesses. Try not to
judge yourself. Simply try to be honest.

» Family and Friends

**Family dinners are a wonderful place to begin wellness-oriented and bal-
anced meals.** Today, plan a family dinner that contains mostly vegetables, a
reasonable serving size of protein (like a lean meat), and a small serving of whole
grains (rice, barley, whole-wheat pasta).

» Nutrition

**Healthy food, especially when you use fresh ingredients and healthy spices,
does not need to taste bad.** Today, make a meal using fresh vegetables, healthy
fats, and lean proteins. Don't forget to season it with some fresh herbs!

Evening Wrap-up

In various ways, we are often told to "buck up." We think that if we just have enough faith, we could overcome whatever obstacle is standing in our way, including depression. But the truth is, whereas depression is a vulnerability, it is *not* a defect of character, and it is not something we can defeat. Paul embraces his strengths and his weaknesses.

We, too, might learn to embrace our vulnerability, to acknowledge our own strengths, and to live with the balance.

If I must boast, I will boast of the things that show my weakness. The God and Father of the Lord Jesus, who is to be praised forever, knows that I am not lying. In Damascus the governor under King Aretas had the city of the Damascenes guarded in order to arrest me. But I was lowered in a basket from a window in the wall and slipped through his hands.

2 CORINTHIANS 11:30–33

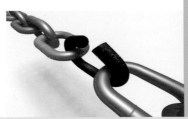

God in our midst, give me the wisdom to see the balance of strength in myself. In Your holy name, Amen.

Morning Reflection

Sometimes managing depression means finding hope that tomorrow will be better. Hope can offer us balance even in the midst of despair. When we can hold on to hope, then we know that tomorrow we can feel differently. Hope can give us the perseverance we need to take today for what it is and tomorrow for what it might be. Today, we will turn our focus to holding on to hope and letting that hope balance our despair.

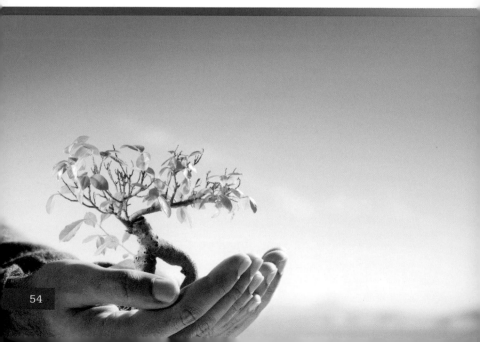

»Faith Life

Today, take ten minutes and write in your journal about a time when you have experienced hope. What did it feel like? Do you think you could find that feeling again?

»Medical

Your physician cannot treat what you do not tell her or him. Make sure that if you have any concerns, tell your doctor. Do not risk your health because you are feeling embarrassed.

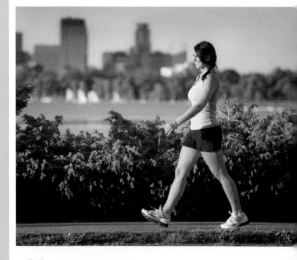

{ Hope can offer us balance even in the midst of despair. }

»Movement

While it can often be easier to sit on the couch, it is often the case that if you are having a bad day, your mood can be lifted by getting some exercise. Try going for a brisk walk today. Remember to stretch afterward!

» Work

When work becomes topsy-turvy, it can be very easy to stress-eat without even recognizing what you are doing. Today, if you start to feel overwhelmed at work, don't head for the vending machines, head for the door! Take a short break outside, breathe in some fresh air, and let your body relax before getting back to work.

» Emotional

Have you seen a counselor or therapist? If not, call and make an appointment. Seeing a professional, even occasionally, can help immensely in managing depression. When you do see someone, the emotional inventories you take every week can help give some insight as to where you stand emotionally.

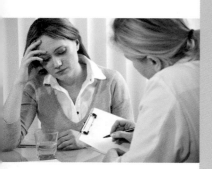

» Family and Friends

Loved ones can offer us perspective and hope, even when we can't seem to find it ourselves. If you are having a bad day, call someone who will listen to you and offer you some perspective.

» Nutrition

If you want to have dessert, instead of a sugary treat, try some fresh fruit served with ricotta cheese or a piece of dark chocolate. Remember, the healthier the food you take in, the better you will feel!

Evening Wrap-up

"Set your hope fully on the grace

to be given you." As we continue on the journey to wellness, we will experience good days and bad days. It is completely normal to experience lows. But when we experience bad days, we can balance the bad by hoping for a better day tomorrow. Hope means that we can both experience the bad while looking forward to better things to come.

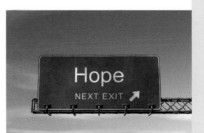

Therefore, with minds that are alert and fully sober, set your hope on the grace to be brought to you when Jesus Christ is revealed at his coming. As obedient children, do not conform to the evil desires you had when you lived in ignorance. But just as he who called you is holy, so be holy in all you do; for it is written: "Be holy, because I am holy."

1 PETER 1:13–16

Loving God, You offer me hope in Your grace. Grant me the perspective to find the hope that You offer, especially on my bad days. In Your holy name, Amen.

Morning Reflection

Congratulations! We have made it to the end of the second week! It is a day for celebration and reflection as we conclude one step on the journey and begin yet another. As we move forward, it is important to take the time to celebrate our victories even while looking forward to the next steps. Today, we will pause to celebrate getting to this point, and we will look forward to the weeks to come.

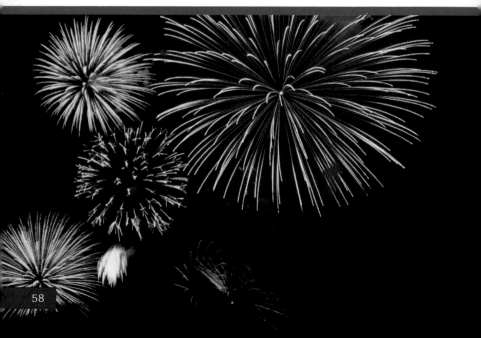

»Faith Life

Much of our faith life is rooted in music. Today, think of a favorite song or hymn and hum a few bars to yourself, or sing aloud while taking a shower or making dinner. Explore the joy of music and the celebration of song!

{ It is a day for celebration and reflection as we conclude one step on the journey and begin yet another. }

»Medical

Refilling prescriptions can be difficult to remember. But it is crucial to maintaining your overall wellness. If your pharmacy has an automatic refill program, take advantage of it. This way, you will never run out of your medication.

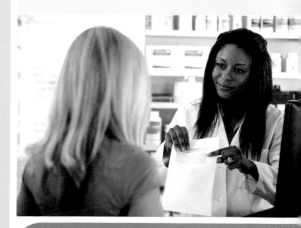

»Movement

Even small amounts of movement can change your body's metabolic balance. If you are waiting in line today, spend time rising up on your toes and relaxing back down. This helps to strengthen your calf muscles, which will help build walking endurance.

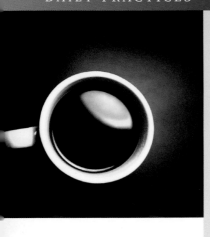

»Work

Caffeine gives you a false energy boost followed by a crash and dehydration. Today, instead of drinking a caffeinated drink throughout the day (such as coffee, tea, or soda), try drinking an herbal tea or even just water to maintain your energy level.

»Emotional

Depression can often make us feel hesitant to celebrate. Today, take five minutes and write in your journal about how you feel celebrating at the end of these two weeks. Does celebrating feel awkward? Does it feel good?

»Family and Friends

Celebrate completing two weeks by trying a new recipe with your family or some friends for a healthy dinner. Try to incorporate mostly vegetables with a lean protein (such as chicken, fish, or tofu) and a serving of whole grains (such as brown rice, quinoa, or whole-wheat pasta).

»Nutrition

Do not drink your calories! Soda, sweetened iced tea, energy drinks, flavored milk, and even "health" drinks such as juices contain a lot of sugar. That sugar can cause your energy to spike and then crash. Try drinking unsweetened tea or seltzer water instead of a sweet drink.

Evening Wrap-up

Weariness and tiredness are a natural part of the journey. Today, after two weeks on the journey, we might be feeling some of that weariness without necessarily feeling the sense of accomplishment. And so, celebrating can be very difficult. But keep in mind the words of Isaiah, "Those who hope in the Lord will renew their strength. They will soar on wings like eagles." God celebrates with us.

Do you not know? Have you not heard? The LORD is the everlasting God, the Creator of the ends of the earth. He will not grow tired or weary, and his understanding no one can fathom. He gives strength to the weary and increases the power of the weak. . . . But those who hope in the LORD will renew their strength. They will soar on wings like eagles; they will run and not grow weary, they will walk and not be faint.

ISAIAH 40:28–29, 31

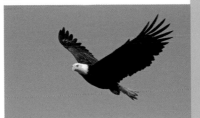

God of joy, help me to celebrate today and to look forward to the coming weeks. Thank You for walking this journey with me. In Your holy name, Amen.

Greg was diagnosed with clinical depression about twenty years ago. Since he was diagnosed, he

has been on a series of antidepressant medications. Some of them have worked better than others over the years. "There were a couple of years where I wasn't really depressed, in the classical sense, but I was always sleeping. I would wake up, go to work, come home, and fall asleep on the couch. Then the next day, it would start all over again. I could function, but just barely."

Then about eight years ago, after having spent several years feeling constantly sleepy, his primary care physician told him that he needed to start an exercise regimen. "I was pre-diabetic and my blood pressure wasn't looking too good, either, so I thought it was a good idea." He came to the Church Health Center.

He started exercising on a regular basis and took a couple of cooking classes, where he learned ways to prepare foods that were lower in fat and higher in nutrients. He soon found, much to his surprise, that his energy started to return. After talking to a counselor about his sleepiness, Greg talked to his doctor and started adjusting his medications so that he would not feel so tired all the time.

Greg is still on a cocktail of medications to help him manage his depression. But he is also exercising nearly every day and eating well. By focusing not just on his depression but on his overall wellness, Greg has found that he feels better and healthier.

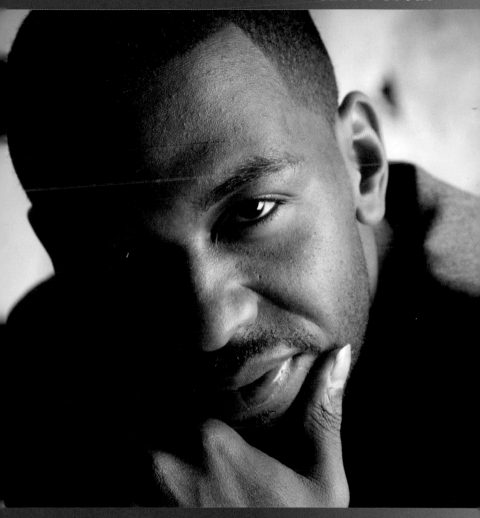

By focusing not just on his depression but on his overall wellness, Greg has found that he feels better and healthier.

Morning Reflection

When managing depression, it can be difficult to get the rest we need. We might find ourselves sleeping all the time and never feeling rested. Alternatively, we might have a difficult time sleeping at all. Either way, managing depression requires paying special attention to both the amount and the quality of our rest. Our overall wellness depends not just on our activity but on our rest. So this week, we will turn our focus to finding ways to get the rest that we need.

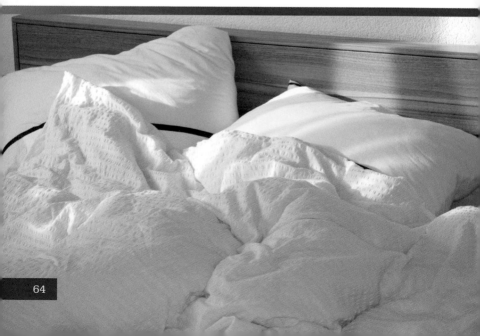

»Faith Life

When you are getting ready for bed at night, having a routine that includes prayer can be very helpful. Tonight, take a minute or two before you go to sleep to pray.

»Medical

What are your sleep patterns? Do you sleep a lot (more than ten hours a night)? Do you have trouble staying asleep? Trouble getting to sleep? Write down your sleep patterns to discuss with your doctor at your next appointment.

{ Our overall wellness depends not just on our activity but on our rest. }

»Movement

Getting some exercise an hour or two before you go to bed can help you relax and get more rejuvenating sleep at night. This evening, go for a short walk and then do some stretching about two hours before you plan on going to bed.

»Work

If you notice that you are having difficulty sleeping at night or getting out of bed in the morning, pay special attention to what you are taking in at work. Lots of sugar? Caffeine? Instead of snacking on unhealthy options, try bringing some herbal tea and cut vegetables for snacks.

»Emotional

When you are sleep deprived, how does it affect your emotional state? Are you irritable? Distracted? Today, take ten minutes to write about how you feel when you do not get enough sleep.

»Family and Friends

Getting rest does not always mean sleeping. It can also mean relaxing and letting down your guard. Today, spend some time relaxing with your family and/or friends.

»Nutrition

Do you have a nighttime snack between dinner and bedtime? Instead of eating carbohydrate-heavy snacks (such as chips or popcorn), try eating some fresh fruit and drinking some chamomile tea. This will keep you from getting a sugar spike right before bed and will help your body to calm.

Evening Wrap-up

We all need rest. Most of us need at least seven or eight hours of sleep every night to function at our best. But in addition to physical sleep, we need spiritual rest. We all carry burdens—it is a part of being human. But in this passage from the Gospel of Matthew, we are assured that Jesus will give us rest.

"All things have been committed to me by my Father. No one knows the Son except the Father, and no one knows the Father except the Son and those to whom the Son chooses to reveal him. Come to me, all you who are weary and burdened, and I will give you rest. Take my yoke upon you and learn from me, for I am gentle and humble in heart, and you will find rest for your souls. For my yoke is easy and my burden is light."

MATTHEW 11:27–30

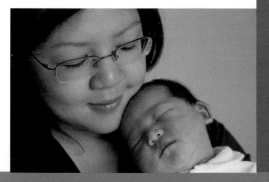

Loving God, help me to lay down my burden, and give me rest. In Your holy name, Amen.

Morning Reflection

Most often, we think of rest as physical sleep: taking a nap or sleeping at night. But rest comes in many different forms. As Greg's story teaches us, we can get lots of sleep and still not be rested. We can find ourselves sleeping constantly and never feeling rested, for a whole host of reasons: spiritual, emotional, and physical. So today, we will focus on how to find ways to rest that do not include sleeping.

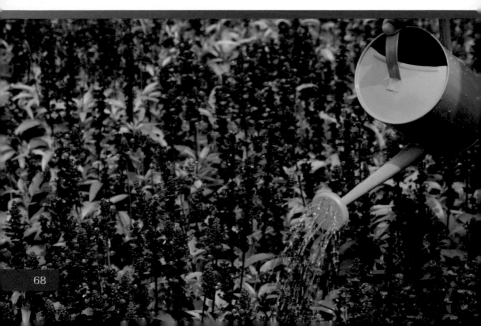

»Faith Life

When we consider "faith life," we often think of our actions. Today, spend ten minutes in quiet meditation. Try to visualize "resting" your spirit.

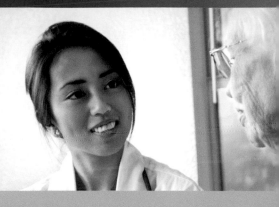

»Medical

Some prescription medications can cause persistent drowsiness as a side effect. If you are taking a number of prescription medications and are constantly sleepy, talk to your doctor. He or she may be able to work with you to adjust your doses and brands so that you feel less tired.

»Movement

When we do not get enough exercise, we can end up feeling lethargic. Today, go for a walk and get your heart rate up. By incorporating regular exercise into your lifestyle, you will have more energy.

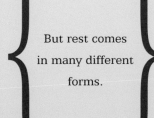

But rest comes in many different forms.

» Work

If you have repetitive work, spending a lot of time in front of a computer, for example, you might find yourself feeling sleepy in the middle of the day. To break up your day a bit, try taking a break to stand up and stretch at least once an hour.

» Emotional

One physical response to stress is sleepiness. Our body tries to just go to sleep when we feel overwhelmed. Today, spend five minutes breathing deeply. Breathe in through your nose and out through your mouth. You may find yourself feeling more energized after you have taken time to breathe.

» Family and Friends

While personal relationships are absolutely important to wellness, it is also important to know your own limits and boundaries. Make sure today that you have some time (even ten minutes) to be by yourself.

» Nutrition

When we eat diets that are high in sugar and fat, our energy levels can be all over the place. Today, when you have a snack, try to eat a protein-rich snack such as some yogurt or nuts. This will help you to have a consistent level of energy throughout the day.

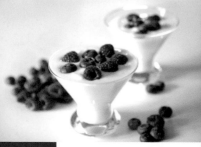

Evening Wrap-up

We might know the story of the hemorrhaging woman and the grace that Jesus showed her. But what we do not often think of is the relief that she must have felt when her bleeding stopped. When we live day-in and day-out with a persistent illness or burden, we can find ourselves feeling desperate and feel enormous relief and rest when that burden is lifted. As we continue on this journey toward wellness, we will experience the lifting of burdens that have long plagued us.

And a woman was there who had been subject to bleeding for twelve years, but no one could heal her. She came up behind him and touched the edge of his cloak, and immediately her bleeding stopped. . . . Then he said to her, "Daughter, your faith has healed you. Go in peace."

Luke 8:43–44, 47–48

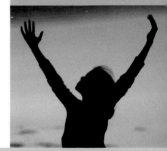

God of healing, help me to identify where I need relief and rest. In Your holy name, Amen.

Morning Reflection

Sometimes to find rest, we need to carve out places and time for ourselves so that we can get rest. That can mean advocating for ourselves and asking for space and time when we need it. But when we are managing depression, it can be very difficult to even recognize when we need that space, let alone actually ask for it. Today, we will turn our focus on how to be advocates for ourselves and how to carve out space to care for ourselves.

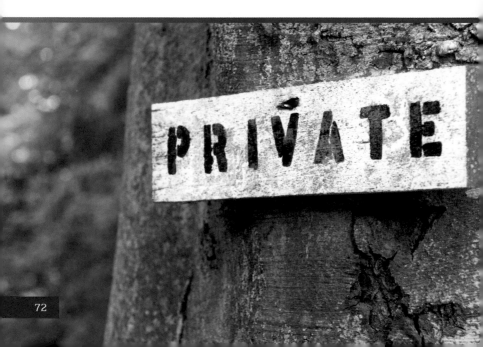

» Faith Life

Is there a place where you feel especially connected to God, for example, your church or an outdoor park? Today, block out some time to spend at this special place.

» Medical

It is Important that you become an advocate for yourself in the medical field. Many people take prescription medications without knowing what they are meant to do. If that describes you, call your doctor's office and ask. It is important that you know why you are taking each of your medications.

» Movement

Combine getting exercise with getting things done by spending some time doing yard work or housework. Moving furniture or planting a garden can give you quite a workout along with a sense of accomplishment.

» Work

Many of us have small tasks at work that get put off day after day. Today, make a list of several small tasks and spend an hour getting them done. Cross each task off as you accomplish it.

» Emotional

Today, take a hot bath. Play some music, let the warm water soak your muscles, and breathe in the steam. It is important to take time for yourself to relax and rest.

» Family and Friends

Today, spend some time with your family and/or friends doing something you really enjoy. Watch a funny movie together, go to the park, or go for a walk.

» Nutrition

If you go out to eat at a restaurant, do not hesitate to request a doggie bag with your dinner. Then you can box up half of your portion before you eat. You are then more likely to eat a healthy portion and less likely to overeat.

In you, Lord, I have taken refuge; let me never be put to shame. In your righteousness, rescue me and deliver me; turn your ear to me and save me. Be my rock of refuge, to which I can always go. . . . For you have been my hope, Sovereign Lord, my confidence since my youth. From birth I have relied on you; you brought me forth from my mother's womb. I will ever praise you.

PSALM 71:1–3, 5–6

Evening Wrap-up

We all need to find a refuge and

safe space to get rest, as illustrated perfectly in this passage from Psalms. But it is not always easy to take that refuge, even when it is offered to us, particularly when we are managing depression. God may give us refuge, as God gave the psalmist refuge, but if we refuse to advocate for ourselves, then we will never get the rest we need.

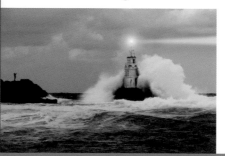

Comforting Lord, thank You for being my refuge. Give me the strength to get the rest I need. In Your holy name, Amen.

Morning Reflection

Most of us are not used to being intentional about getting rest. After all, we live in a "Go! Go! Go!" culture, where productivity tends to be valued more than anything. But the consequence of the constant motion is that our overall wellness suffers. Our bodies and our spirits need time for rejuvenation and rest. This is particularly true when we are managing depression. Today, we will focus on how to slow down even when the rest of the world seems to be pushing us to move forward.

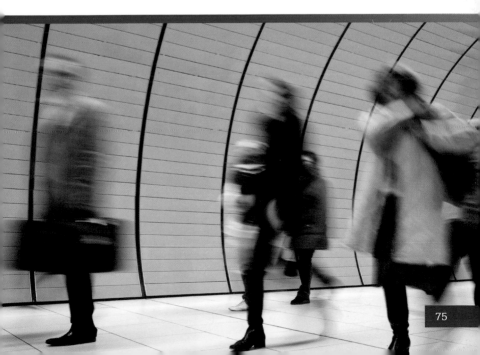

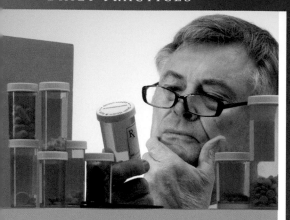

»Faith Life

Today, go for a walking meditation. Go for a slow walk, focusing on your movements and your breath, one step at a time. Remember that God created your body and the air that you are breathing.

»Medical

When was the last time you cleaned out your medicine cabinet? Lots of accidents can be avoided by disposing of expired and old medication. Today take inventory of your medicine cabinet and throw out anything expired or unusable.

»Movement

Today, take ten minutes and do some stretching. Be sure to warm up your muscles a bit and then breathe into the stretches. Stretch your back, arms, and legs.

{ Go for a slow walk, focusing on your movements and your breath, one step at a time. }

»Work

Do you work in a fast-paced environment? If so, find a place where you can step outside the action, if only for a minute, to catch your breath and find your center before returning to work.

»Emotional

Sometimes, we can feel pulled in seventeen different directions at the same time. To pull yourself together and feel whole, take a shower, let yourself relax, and breathe before getting back to your life.

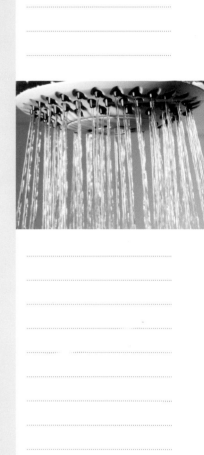

»Family and Friends

Tonight, enjoy an evening out with your family or friends. Go to a healthy restaurant, and try something on the menu that you may not have had otherwise.

»Nutrition

Do you eat fast? Many of us have gotten into the habit of wolfing down our food the instant it hits the plate in front of us. Today, slow down, take one bite at a time, and pay attention. When you stop feeling hungry, stop eating.

Evening Wrap-up

Thus the heavens and the earth were completed in all their vast array. By the seventh day God had finished the work he had been doing; so on the seventh day he rested from all his work. Then God blessed the seventh day and made it holy, because on it he rested from all the work of creating that he had done.

GENESIS 2:1–3

It is difficult to get adequate rest,

especially in our culture of constant motion. However, even God took the time to rest on the seventh day. We · need to learn how to take time to slow down, breathe, and reflect as we continue on the journey toward wellness. Learning how to rest can be one of the most difficult lessons any of us will learn, but it can also be one of the most important on this journey.

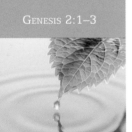

Loving and merciful God, help me to find rest in You. Give me the courage to face stillness and rest. In Your holy name, Amen.

Morning Reflection

Sometimes getting adequate rest means realizing when we need to allow others to care for us. In our first week on this journey, we acknowledged that reaching out is important. It is also important to accept help and to ask for it when we need it. In asking for help and allowing others to care for us, we can get the rest that our bodies and spirits so desperately need.

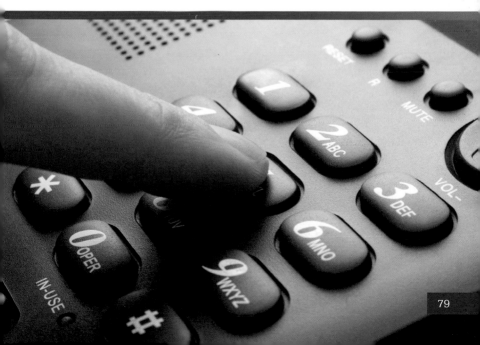

» Faith Life

Yesterday you spent time in a walking meditation. Today, spend ten minutes sitting quietly in meditation. Try to quiet your mind and clear out the clutter, stress, and anxiety. Breathe and let in God.

» Medical

Remember that medications can have side effects—some are physical and some are emotional. If you are having emotional side effects (such as increased depression, anxiety, or euphoria) or physical side effects (such as weight gain, hunger, or a rash), let your doctor know as soon as possible.

» Movement

Put on some music. Spend five minutes today dancing to the music in whatever way you can dance. Move your whole body as much as you can. Move your head, your back, your fingers, your toes. Feel your entire body working together.

» Work

Wherever you work, find a convenient place where you can keep some healthy snacks on hand. When you take a break, instead of going to a vending machine, enjoy a healthy snack and a short walk.

» Emotional

Today, take an emotional inventory. Has the focus on rest changed your perspective at all? Compare this week's inventory to last week's. How are things different? What has remained the same?

» Family and Friends

Do you allow your family to care for you? Do you ever ask your friends for help? Recruit some of your family and friends to help you clean out your kitchen. Throw out expired foods as well as processed foods with a high sugar or fat content.

» Nutrition

Move the unhealthy snacks, such as potato chips or cookies, out of reach. Set them on a high shelf in the pantry or throw them out entirely. Move healthy snacks, such as fresh vegetables or fruits, into easy-to-grab places.

Evening Wrap-up

Have you ever muttered the phrase

"I'll just do it myself!"? So often we find it is easier to just take up a burden on our own than to rely on someone else. Putting trust in another means opening ourselves up to the possibility of disappointment, hurt, and loss of control. But when managing depression, it is very important to rely on other people. Remember the words of the psalmist, "He refreshes my soul."

The LORD is my shepherd, I lack nothing. He makes me lie down in green pastures, he leads me beside quiet waters, he refreshes my soul. He guides me along the right paths for his name's sake. Even though I walk through the darkest valley, I will fear no evil, for you are with me; your rod and your staff, they comfort me.

PSALM 23:1–4

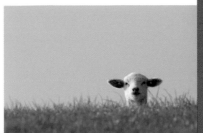

Loving God, grant me rest and restore my soul. Help me to reach out and accept help when I need it. In Your holy name, Amen.

Morning Reflection

Getting adequate rest is more than just "not doing anything" for a while. Adequate rest is a form of sustenance. Just like food and water, rest is nourishing. It gives us energy and keeps us healthy. Rest is restorative, and we, too often, simply feel that we do not have the time. But the truth is that if we do not make the time, our bodies and spirits suffer. To truly continue on this journey toward wellness, we must learn how to rest.

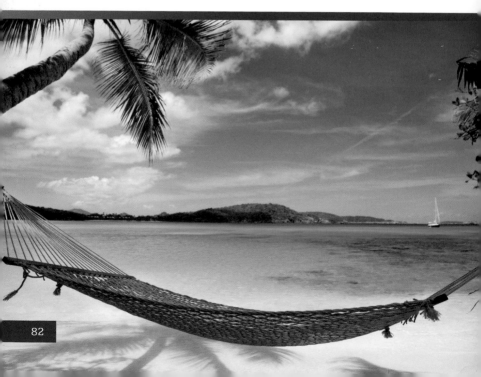

»Faith Life

When you pray, do you also have your to-do list running through your head? Today, take five minutes to pray, but first try to sit and quiet yourself. Find your center and let your prayer fill your whole spirit.

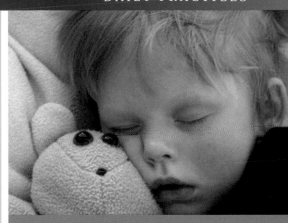

»Medical

Sleeping is not just something that is enjoyable or helpful. Proper rest is crucial to our physical health and an important part of processing stress. When we consistently lack sleep, we can become sleep deprived. Today, read up on sleep deprivation and commit to getting a full night's sleep.

»Movement

Today, do thirty jumping jacks, and then stretch out your arms and back. Doing even a small amount of exercise can give you the energy you need to get through the rest of your day.

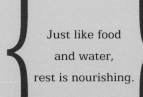

{ Just like food and water, rest is nourishing. }

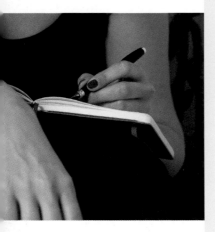

» Work

Having a difficult day at work? Instead of focusing on the negative, think of something fun that you can do when you get home, even if it is simply getting outside to enjoy the fresh air. Write it down in a place where you can see your plans for your evening.

» Emotional

When we do not take the time to enjoy ourselves, we can become overwhelmed. Today spend five minutes writing in your journal about the things that you enjoy doing.

» Family and Friends

Our personal relationships feed our spirits in the same way that healthy food feeds our bodies. Today, make a list of the ways that the important personal relationships in your life feed you.

» Nutrition

Choosing a wellness-oriented diet is all about sustenance. Today, cook a delicious and healthy meal for yourself, such as whole-grain pasta, or lean meat with steamed vegetables. Eating well helps us feel better and can really help us keep a positive attitude.

Evening Wrap-up

Rest is sustenance, in the same way that food is sustenance. We cannot live and be well without rest. On our journey to wellness, learning to balance rest with everything else in our lives is just like learning to cook different meals or exercising. It takes time and effort. But as we walk on the journey, we can rest in the assurance that, even as we struggle, God walks with us and sustains us. The psalmist assures us that the reason we wake in the morning is because the Lord sustains us. What a blessing!

I lie down and sleep; I wake again, because the LORD sustains me. I will not fear though tens of thousands assail me on every side. Arise, LORD! Deliver me, my God! . . . From the LORD comes deliverance. May your blessing be on your people.

PSALM 3:5–8

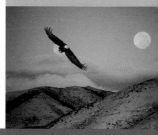

Heavenly Father, thank You for sustaining me on this journey. Help me as I continue to take steps toward wellness. In Your holy name, Amen.

Morning Reflection

Congratulations! Another week completed! We have now officially reached the halfway point of this particular six-week journey. Today is a day for (restful) celebrations! But sometimes a halfway point can feel both exciting and discouraging. We can look back at the progress we have made so far, while also feeling like we still have to travel a great distance. As much as possible, let us make today a celebration of how far we have come, and a preparation for the steps we have yet to take.

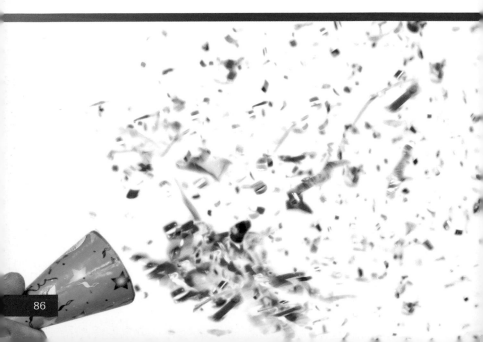

»Faith Life

Look back at your description of your faith life during the first week of this journey. How would you describe your faith life now? What has changed?

»Medical

Many people with clinical or severe depression do not have typical symptoms. If you experience any combination of these symptoms for more than three weeks, talk to your doctor: headaches, aches and pains, unexplained digestive trouble, change in appetite, or a drastic change in weight.

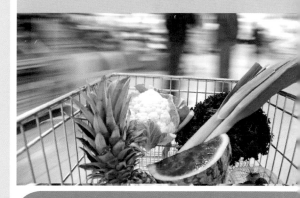

»Movement

When you go to the grocery store, once you have loaded up your cart, take an extra walk around the store. It won't take you much time, and it will add another hundred or so steps to your day (depending on the size of your grocery store!).

{ Today is a day for (restful) celebrations! }

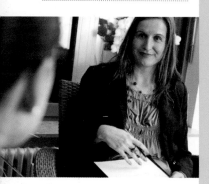

»Work

Good posture helps you to breathe, increases strength in your back and abdomen, and can help decrease back pain and headaches. Today at work, try to remind yourself to keep your head up and your shoulders back and relaxed.

»Emotional

If you have not seen a counselor or a therapist, now is the perfect time to call. Remember, a counselor can give you great perspective on how to manage your own personal struggle with depression.

»Family and Friends

If you are sharing this journey with some friends and family members, have a celebratory dinner tonight with them. Either cook at home or choose a healthy-menu restaurant where you can celebrate and be celebrated.

»Nutrition

Celebrate with something sweet! Try fresh fruit, like pineapple or raspberries, with some yogurt, or a banana with a small bite of dark chocolate.

Evening Wrap-up

We are reminded many times throughout the Bible to keep the Sabbath, to keep a day of rest. Observing a Sabbath can be a way of celebrating all that we have done. Keep in mind that God rested on the seventh day and that God created the Sabbath for us. Today, let us sit back and take in the progress that we have made on this journey, rest, and prepare for the next steps.

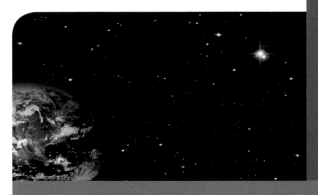

"Remember the Sabbath day by keeping it holy. Six days you shall labor and do all your work, but the seventh day is a sabbath to the Lord your God. On it you shall not do any work, neither you, nor your son or daughter, nor your male or female servant, nor your animals, nor any foreigner residing in your towns. For in six days the Lord made the heavens and the earth, the sea, and all that is in them, but he rested on the seventh day. Therefore the Lord blessed the Sabbath day and made it holy."

Exodus 20:8–11

Sustaining Lord, thank You for walking with me on this journey. Help me to prepare for the next steps. In Your holy name, Amen.

Michael has struggled with depression since he was a teenager. When he was in college, he often had difficulty focusing. He started using alcohol as a way to cope. For many years he used alcohol and food as self-medication. "I figured if I couldn't feel good, then feeling nothing was a good alternative."

He gained weight and gradually settled into a more sedentary lifestyle. "Why bother trying to exercise or anything like that? It never made me feel better."

But one day he went to the doctor and got a wake-up call. He was showing early signs of heart disease. His doctor recommended that he look into joining the Church Health Center to get his nutritional and exercise needs addressed. But he found counselors at the Church Health Center as well. "My counselor really helped me to see that I was not lazy or a bum but that I was really struggling with depression."

Michael did not want to take medication to treat his depression, so he and his counselor figured out a regimen that helps him manage his depression without a prescription. "I take some herbal supplements every day. I quit drinking alcohol altogether. And I exercise and eat well every day." In addition to taking care of his physical needs, Michael has discovered a newfound love of volunteering. "When I took the time to heal myself, I also found the time to reach out to people who were really in need," he said.

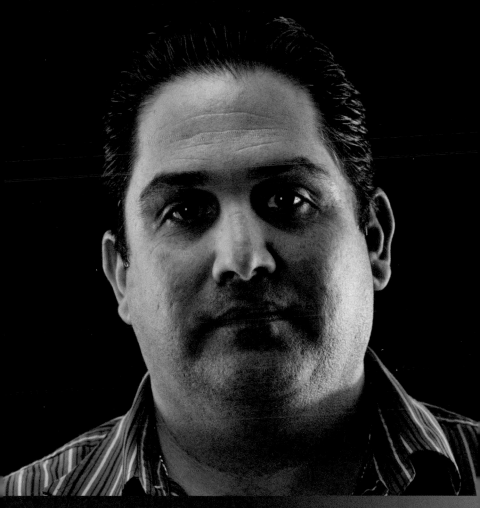

"When I took the time to heal myself,
I also found the time to reach out to
people who were really in need."

Depression

Morning Reflection

We have arrived at the fourth week of our six-week journey, and we may be starting to feel a difference from where we started. But no matter how far we have come, there will probably always be a part of us that wishes for someone to snap their fingers and make us better. We want to feel better and *right now*. Healing, for better or for worse, is a long process. And this week, we will focus on what the healing process means for managing our depression.

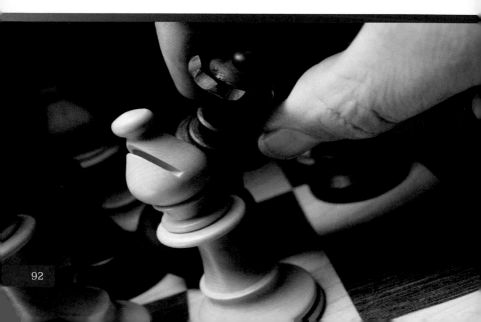

»Faith Life

Have you ever experienced God's healing grace? When? Today, write in your journal about what God's healing has meant to you. Remember that God's healing comes in many different forms.

»Medical

Are you on medications? Have you been feeling better? Do not stop taking any medications until you have discussed it with your primary care provider. Stopping medication suddenly can lead to relapse, drug resistance, or unexpected side effects.

»Movement

Now that we are a few weeks in, think about what new kinds of exercise you might want to do. Do you like dance, yoga, or Zumba? Maybe you want to challenge yourself to walking a 5K or joining a pool? Try to think of activities you like to do—or perhaps, that you *used* to like—and how they might enhance your exercise.

{ Healing, for better or for worse, is a long process. }

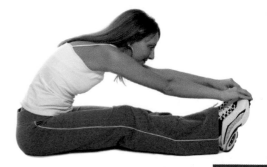

93

»Work

If you find yourself standing in one place for a period of time (making copies, talking on the phone, waiting for lunch to heat up), spend that time raising yourself onto your toes and then lowering yourself back down, increasing the strength in your calves.

»Emotional

Today, spend five minutes writing in your journal about what healing means for you on this journey. Do you want to feel happy? Start enjoying something that you've lost enjoyment for.

»Family and Friends

A very important part of the healing process in managing depression is becoming a part of the community. If you do not have a built-in community (as in a church or school), try joining a book club or similar interest group.

»Nutrition

When "low-fat," "reduced-sugar," and "light" versions of your staple foods are available, choose them over the full-fat, full-sugar versions. But don't be fooled—just because something is low-fat doesn't mean it's healthy. Be aware of advertising gimmicks and make the best choices you can.

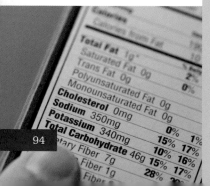

Evening Wrap-up

We all have heard the miraculous stories of Jesus healing.

But one of the highlights of this particular healing story is what happens after the Gerasene demoniac is healed; Jesus sends him back into the community. Jesus begins the healing process, and sends the man back into the community so that he can continue the journey. Like this man, we must continue with the healing even once we are feeling better.

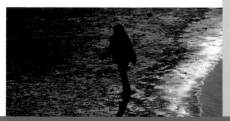

They sailed to the region of the Gerasenes . . . When Jesus stepped ashore, he was met by a demon-possessed man from the town. . . . The demons begged Jesus to let them go into the pigs, and he gave them permission. . . . The man from whom the demons had gone out begged to go with him, but Jesus sent him away, saying, "Return home and tell how much God has done for you." So the man went away and told all over town how much Jesus had done for him.

LUKE 8:26–27, 32, 38–39

God of the long journeys, help me to see Your healing hand in my life. In Your holy name, Amen.

Morning Reflection

Healing is a gradual process. It is a journey. And because it is a journey, it can sometimes include setbacks. The important thing is to continue moving forward even when we experience a setback. Progress and healing does not always happen in one direction. Instead, we might take a couple of steps forward, one step back, maybe even a step or two sideways. The journey to wellness is circuitous at times. Today, we will focus on the roundabout journey to healing and wellness.

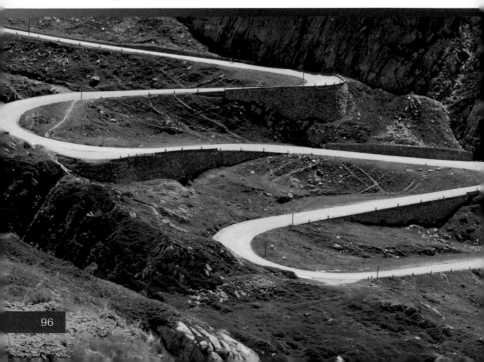

»Faith Life

Today, reflect on a time when you experienced a setback in your faith life. Take five minutes and write in your journal about how that setback changed your faith journey.

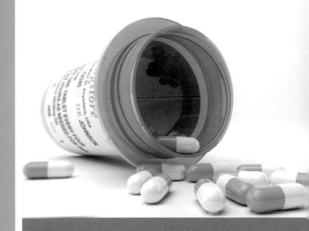

»Medical

If you forget to take your medication for one dose, do not take a double dose. Instead, call your primary care provider and ask whether you should take a dose immediately, or wait until it is time for the next dose to get back on track.

{ Progress and healing does not always happen in one direction. }

»Movement

Spend ten minutes walking around your house (or walk around your neighborhood, if you feel comfortable) taking two steps forward and one step backward. Notice that you still move forward. Also, walking backward exercises different muscles than walking forward.

» Work

How has this journey impacted your work life thus far? Have you noticed changes in your attitude, your work ethic, and/or your productivity? Consider how you have changed your work life today and take note of your improvements.

» Emotional

Managing depression is a rocky terrain. Take five minutes today and write about how setbacks make you feel. How have you coped in the past? How would you like to cope with them in the future?

» Family and Friends

We can have setbacks in our relation-ships that affect our depression. Today, write a letter to a person whom you want to make amends with. Drop it in the mail if you wish, or just hold on to it yourself and think about how you might take the first step toward reconciliation.

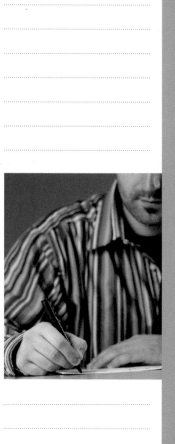

» Nutrition

Nutritional setbacks happen. We give in to the temptation of a doughnut or eat too much out at a friend's birthday dinner. The temptation is to starve yourself the day after to "make up" for the setback. Instead, just get back on track eating a healthy and reasonable diet.

Evening Wrap-up

Healing happens in a roundabout way. On days when we are feeling better, or even feel completely healed, we can still experience unexpected turns in the road that might knock us off course. Consider the man Jesus healed in this story. Jesus healed his eyesight, but then he had to continue his life—he had an entire story after his initial healing that we never know. He probably had good days and bad, and through all that, God walked that journey with him, just as God walks our journey with us.

Some people brought a blind man and begged Jesus to touch him. He took the blind man by the hand and led him outside the village. When he had spit on the man's eyes and put his hands on him . . .his eyes were opened, his sight was restored, and he saw everything clearly. Jesus sent him home.

MARK 8:22–23, 25–26

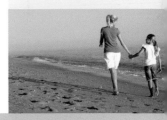

Loving God, thank You for walking this journey with me. Help me to persevere even when I get knocked off course. In Your holy name, Amen.

Morning Reflection

Part of healing is adjusting our attitude—realizing that we are valuable and learning to love and value ourselves. Managing depression is a long journey that requires taking a good hard look at ourselves. So often, depression is linked to a complete lack of self-worth. We think that we are not worth caring for. But the truth is, we are all made in God's image, and we are loved by God. If God finds value in us, then surely we can find the strength to love ourselves.

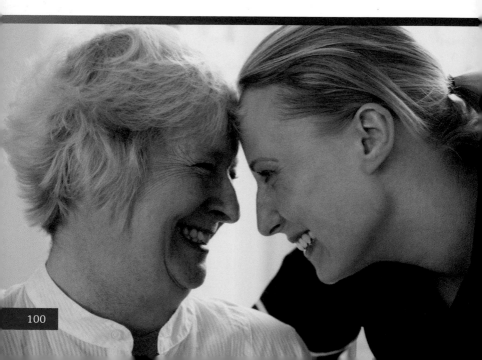

» Faith Life

Do you think of yourself as a person created in the image of God? Take five minutes and write about what you see in yourself that is God-like. Be as specific as possible.

» Medical

It is important to understand wound care and how to recognize if a wound is not healing properly. Wounds should heal more or less within a week. If wounds, particularly on the legs or feet, are not healing quickly, it is important to contact a primary care provider.

» Movement

Today spend ten minutes stretching and exploring all of the parts that God made. Touch your toes, cross your arms over your chest, roll your neck, stretch your arms up over your head, and stretch your back.

» Work

If you must go out for lunch at work, try to avoid eating fast food. Instead, try to find a place where you can order lean protein and vegetables that are not fried.

» Emotional

One of the keys to emotional wellness is to spend time engaged in self-care. Today, write down one area in your life where you could use some more self-care. Do you need to find some extra alone time? Do you need to schedule more time with friends?

» Family and Friends

If you are having a difficult time finding value in yourself, call a friend and ask for some perspective. It might feel awkward at first, but hearing what people who love you love about you can give you a place to focus.

» Nutrition

Using table salt can greatly increase the sodium content of your food. Try using a season substitute, such as garlic *powder* (not garlic salt!). Switch the salt and pepper shakers so that you are more tempted to go straight for the pepper.

> *But now, this is what the LORD says—he who created you, Jacob, he who formed you, Israel: "Do not fear, for I have redeemed you; I have summoned you by name; you are mine. When you pass through the waters, I will be with you; and when you pass through the rivers, they will not sweep over you. When you walk through the fire, you will not be burned; the flames will not set you ablaze. For I am the LORD your God, the Holy One of Israel, your Savior; I give Egypt for your ransom, Cush and Seba in your stead.*
>
> ISAIAH 43:1–3

Evening Wrap-up

Wherever we are on the journey,

and however we are feeling as we walk, God walks with us. God has called each of us by name, and we belong to God. If there is no other reason, that should assure us that we are worthy of care. God cares for us, and so we can care for ourselves and for each other.

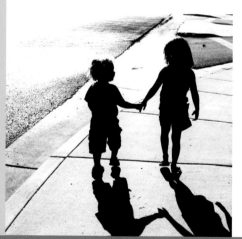

Merciful God, I know that You are with me. Please keep reminding me of Your constant presence on my journey. Amen.

Morning Reflection

We often think of depression as only an emotional problem. The truth is, however, that depression has emotional and physical causes and consequences. This is why managing depression can be so convoluted and difficult. We must balance the work that we do emotionally with our own physical wellness. The journey to wellness cannot be only an emotional journey. Today, we will turn our focus to the physical nature of our journey toward wellness.

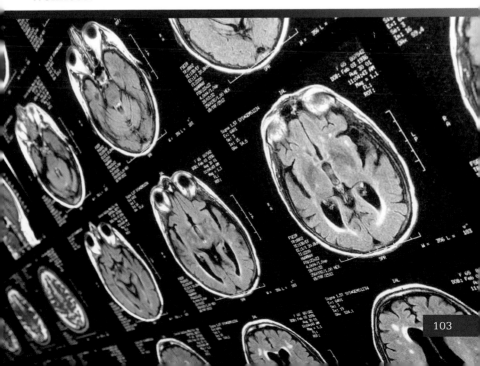

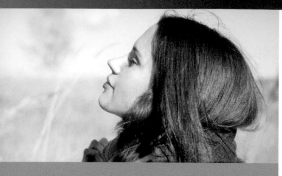

»Medical

While overexposure to sun can be dangerous, a moderate amount of exposure every day can actually be good for you! Today, head outside for fifteen minutes or so to let the sun kiss your face.

»Movement

Today go for a brisk walk, and when you are finished, spend at least five minutes stretching. Try to feel and stretch as many muscles in your body as possible.

»Faith Life

Remember that God came to us as a human—with a body! Today, pray a walking prayer. Go for a walk, concentrate on your body moving, the breath you breathe, the smells you smell, and give thanks for all those aspects of your body.

{ Today, pray a walking prayer. }

»Work

Bring a refillable water bottle to work.
When you are feeling thirsty, or craving a soda, fill up your water bottle and sip from the bottle throughout the day. Staying hydrated will help you keep your energy levels up and will keep you from drinking sugary sodas.

»Emotional

Our emotions are more tied up with our bodies than we usually realize. Today, spend five minutes smiling, even if you do not feel like smiling. Chances are, you will feel a little better at the end of those five minutes.

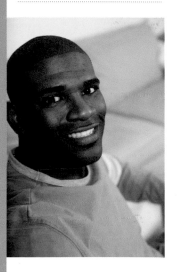

»Family and Friends

Eating or exercising with friends and family can be a great way to keep your wellness goals. Today, think of a friend whom you can set a goal with. Perhaps they have the same goal, or will help hold you accountable to the goals you are setting for yourself.

»Nutrition

Drink about two glasses of milk today.
But instead of whole milk, drink low-fat milk (either 1 percent or skim). Two servings of low-fat dairy each day is an important part of a healthy diet.

Heal me, Lord, and I will be healed; save me and I will be saved, for you are the one I praise. They keep saying to me, "Where is the word of the Lord? Let it now be fulfilled!" I have not run away from being your shepherd; you know I have not desired the day of despair. What passes my lips is open before you.

Jeremiah 17:14–16

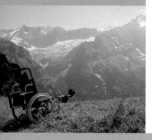

Evening Wrap-up

Keep in mind that God chose to come to us as a human person.

He gave us the precious gift of His own body. Furthermore, while Jesus was on earth, He spent a good deal of time healing bodies in various states of distress. So when Jeremiah calls out to God, "Heal me, Lord, and I will be healed," he means it. On our journey toward wellness, we can find physical healing as well as emotional healing as a part of the process.

Healing God, thank You for caring for my body. Help me on this journey to find healing in my body. Amen.

Morning Reflection

On this journey to wellness, we are working to heal both our bodies and our spirits. While we are often tempted to act like wellness is merely a physical process, we are coming to learn on this journey that wellness means wellness in body and spirit. Managing depression requires both physical healing and spiritual healing. Today, we will turn our focus to the ways that we are working to revive our spirits on this journey.

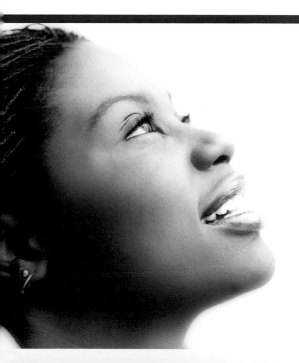

» Faith Life

What does having a healthy spirit mean to you? Today, take some time to pray, and then take five minutes and write in your journal about what a healthy spirit means.

» Medical

If you are physically sick (with a cold or the flu), make sure that you get as much rest as you possibly can. Stay home from work if you are able, and stay in bed. The more you rest, the sooner you will be back to your old self.

» Movement

Helping a neighbor to do yard work or even to move is a wonderful act of kindness and generosity, and it can get your heart rate up and burn calories, to boot! Today, try to help a friend, family member, or neighbor with a project.

» Work

We do not often think of work as something to enjoy. Today find something that you enjoy about being at work, and focus on that. If you cannot think of something, try going for a walk or stepping outside when you have a break.

» Emotional

We often expect perfection of ourselves. The trouble with such expectations is that we are simply not perfect, and we can become demoralized. Today, write for ten minutes about a time when you have expected perfection from yourself.

» Family and Friends

Do your family and friends make you laugh? Laughter is a wonderful way to burn calories and generally lift your mood. Today, when spending time with friends or family, let yourself laugh freely.

» Nutrition

Serving water with meals is a great way to meet your daily water goals (at least eight eight-ounce glasses). Today, serve water instead of soda or other sweetened beverages.

Evening Wrap-up

At this point in our journey, we might be able to see a real difference in our day-to-day lives. The contents of our refrigerator might be different from what they were four weeks ago. We are exercising more regularly. And, hopefully, we are feeling a bit of a lift in our spirits. But realize that even if we do not feel a huge transformation, God continues to hear our cries. God continues to walk the journey with us.

I cried out to God for help; I cried out to God to hear me. When I was in distress, I sought the Lord; at night I stretched out untiring hands, and I would not be comforted. I remembered you, God. . . . My heart meditated and my spirit asked.

PSALM 77:1–3, 6

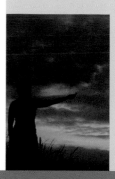

Loving God, help me to heal my spirit as I continue on this journey to wellness. In Your holy name, Amen.

Morning Reflection

Part of the healing process in managing depression

is learning—or re-learning—to experience joy and
happiness. For some of us, this is easier said than done,
but it is important for all of us. After all, God created this
world and us in it, so when we take the time to enjoy the
world, we are taking time to love and enjoy God's creation.
Depression can sometimes hinder our ability to really
experience enjoyment, so today we will focus on ways to
experience enjoyment on the journey to wellness.

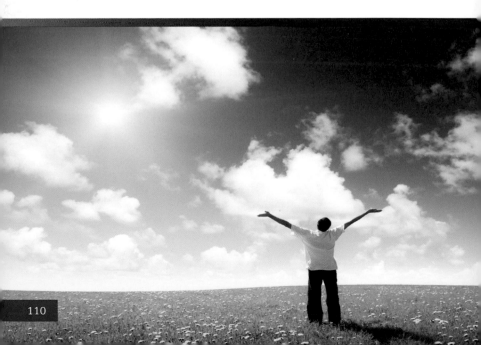

»Faith Life

Prayer and meditation do not always have to be somber and solemn. Laughter and fun can be a part of prayer, just as rejoicing needs to be a part of our faith life. Think of something funny that has happened and thank God for giving us humor in our lives.

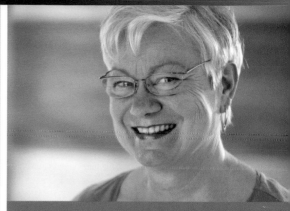

»Medical

Don't be intimidated by the clinic or the hospital. We might think of these places as somber or painful, but clinics are full of medical professionals who enjoy their work and have a good time, even in the midst of painful circumstances. Today, try to remember that your medical team is trying to help you and offer a prayer for success and joy in their work.

{ God created this world and us in it, so when we take the time to enjoy the world, we are taking time to love and enjoy God's creation. }

»Movement

Spend some time today doing something you enjoy. Go for a walk or dance around your house. Having fun while exercising makes it more likely that you will continue exercising.

111

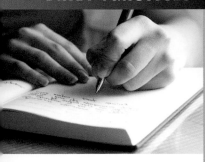

» Work

What are your habits when you get home from work? Do you eat? Clean? Watch television? Pay attention today to the small things that you do. Write down your actions in fifteen-minute increments. You may be surprised!

» Emotional

It is time for another emotional inventory! Write in your journal how you are feeling today and this week. Compare it to the previous three weeks.

» Family and Friends

Personal relationships can offer you encouragement and perspective that you may not have for yourself. Identify two people in your life who are particularly gifted in offering you encouragement when you need it.

» Nutrition

Instead of potato chips and a cream-based dip (like onion dip), try making some salsa and eat it with some baked tortilla chips for a delicious and healthy party snack.

Evening Wrap-up

Enjoyment, though it does not always come easily, is such an important part of our journey that even Paul admonishes us to be joyful. We have been created for rejoicing! But when it is difficult to find the space for enjoyment, we can turn to God. Paul also reminds us that God is faithful to us, and God walks with us, even when we might have a hard time finding joy on the journey.

Rejoice always, pray continually, give thanks in all circumstances; for this is God's will for you in Christ Jesus. Do not quench the Spirit. . . hold on to what is good. . . . May God himself, the God of peace, sanctify you through and through. May your whole spirit, soul and body be kept blameless at the coming of our Lord Jesus Christ. The one who calls you is faithful, and he will do it.

1 THESSALONIANS 5:16–21, 23–24

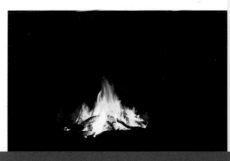

Joyous Lord, help me today to rejoice in Your creation and in myself. In Your holy name, Amen.

Morning Reflection

Even though we are focusing this journey on managing depression, this journey is a path to wellness, and wellness is about wholeness. When we only care for one part of ourselves while we neglect other parts, we do not care for our whole selves. God created us as whole selves—body and spirit—and so we ought to care for the entire self as well. Today, we will focus on ways that we can appreciate and care for our entire self.

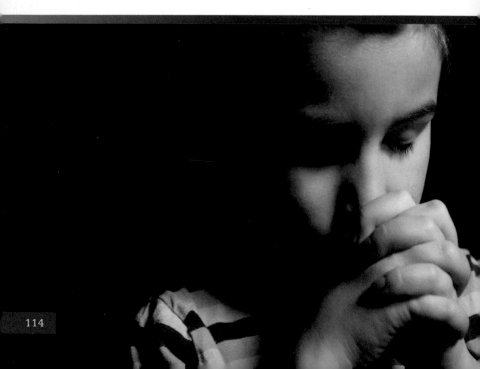

»Faith Life

When you pray today, wiggle your fingers and toes. Stand up and sit down. Jump up and down. Breathe in and out. Think about how our whole bodies can pray, rather than just our minds or our spirits.

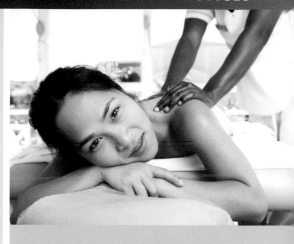

»Medical

Sometimes alternative therapies can help us to manage our depression in a whole-body, wellness-oriented way. Today, try getting a massage for stress release.

»Movement

Go for a walk today. Try to notice how your entire body works together. Then turn your attention outside and try to notice how God's whole creation works together with you in it.

{ Today, we will focus on ways that we can appreciate and care for the self as an entirety. }

115

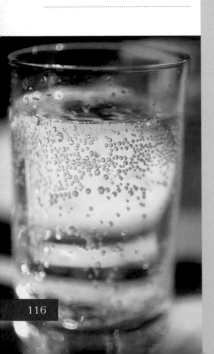

»Work

Most of us work using one aspect of our personality more than other parts. Today, try to take five minutes at work and use another aspect of your body or personality. If you sit at a computer all day, go for a short walk. If you're on the phone, take a moment to stretch, and if you stand all day, find a quiet place to sit.

»Emotional

Do you have trouble enjoying day-to-day activities? If so, make an appointment with a counselor or therapist. A professional can help give you strategies for managing your depression that will be custom-made for you.

»Family and Friends

Often our friends and family are stronger than we know and may be able to help us shoulder even the hardest burdens. Today, think of one trusted friend and share a challenge from your wellness journey. See how they can be a welcome help!

»Nutrition

If you are a soda drinker and just can't give up the habit, try drinking seltzer water for a carbonated treat. If you want something sweet, try adding a small amount of no-sugar-added fruit juice to the seltzer.

Evening Wrap-up

Congratulations! You have reached the end of another week! Our six-week journey is approaching the end, but the journey to wellness will continue even after you have completed this book. As we continue the journey, it is important to keep in mind that we are created whole beings. God has created us whole, and God is our advocate on this journey.

"The Lord is my strength and my defense; he has become my salvation. He is my God, and I will praise him, my father's God, and I will exalt him. The Lord is a warrior; the Lord is his name. Pharaoh's chariots and his army he has hurled into the sea.

Exodus 15:2–4

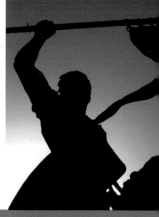

Giving God, bless me with strength and the eyes to see myself as a whole person, created by You. Amen.

Ada grew up with a violent alcoholic father. As

a child, she remembers her mother falling in the living room and her dad trying to kick her. Ada desperately tried to pull him *just a little farther* away so that his foot couldn't reach her mom. Eventually, when Ada was seventeen years old, she ran away from home, taking the family dog with her. After escaping the trauma of her home, Ada sank into a depression that lasted for the next twenty-six years of her life.

Despite her depression, Ada married, had children, and got a job as a nurse. But she struggled. She was on prescription antidepressants and overdosed at one point. She spent some time in a mental hospital. She could not hold down a job. Eventually, her marriage came to an end. She was faced with tragedy after tragedy, and it seemed to her that she would never be happy again.

But after yet another stay in a mental hospital, Ada sought the counsel of a friend who was a professional pastoral counselor at the Church Health Center. Ada started the long, hard work of learning to love herself—for the first time in her life. She is now working as a mental health counselor and has been helping people for the last decade. Asked about her recovery, Ada quotes Joel 2:25, "I will restore to you the years that the locusts have eaten." She continues, "He has restored my life with a vengeance!"

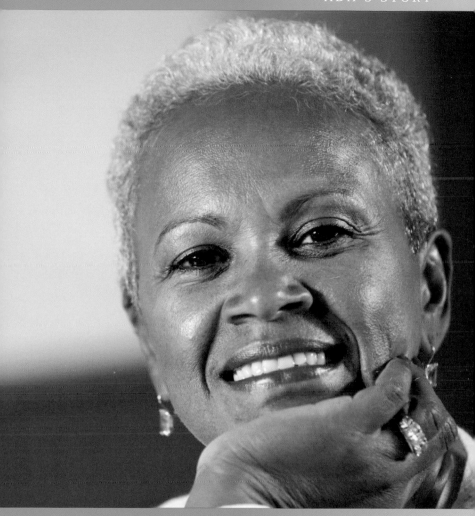

"He has restored my life with a vengeance!"

Depression

Morning Reflection

The journey to wellness is, as we have already seen, a convoluted one at times. It can leave us feeling topsy-turvy. But the journey can also bring us moments of clarity, and at times, we may look back on the journey and see that we have been renewed in the journey. Managing depression is not always just about fighting through the bad times. It is about finding renewal. We can actually become new people. So this week we will focus on how the journey can renew us.

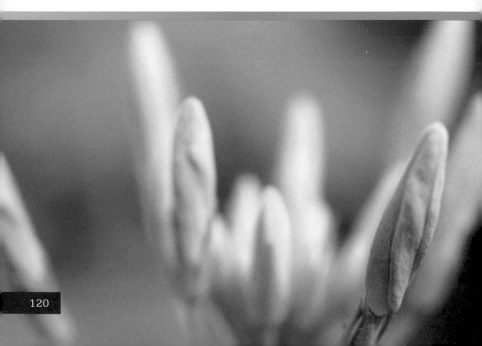

»Faith Life

Remember that Jesus promises us life in abundance. Take five minutes today and write about what you think "abundant life" means. Does this journey to wellness get you closer to your understanding of "abundant life"?

{ It is about finding renewal. }

»Medical

Sometimes starting a new medication can make us feel like a different person. This can sometimes be a good sign, sometimes not. If you have started a new medication and you feel your personality significantly altered, talk with your doctor.

»Movement

Today, go for a walk and take a coin with you. Flip the coin each time you arrive at a corner to determine which direction you will walk. Enjoy the spontaneity of taking a walk without a particular destination.

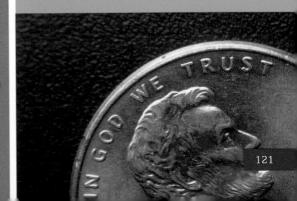

»Work

Instead of going out to eat or getting lunch out of a vending machine, bring in a lunch made from your leftovers from last night's dinner. It is almost guaranteed to be healthier, and it is much less expensive!

»Emotional

The unpredictability of our wellness journey can sometimes feel overwhelming. Today, make a list of what your expectations are at this point in your journey. Compare them with your expectations at the beginning of the journey.

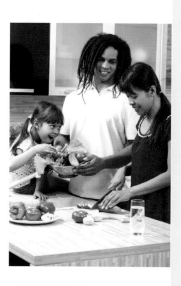

»Family and Friends

Family and friends can be our constants when other things in life are unpredictable. Today, make a healthy meal for your family or some friends. Enjoy the food, but focus on the company and conversation.

»Nutrition

When you are trying to cut out sugar, add lemon, orange, or lime zest to a recipe. The citrus zest will add flavor and interest to a dish, so you will be less likely to miss the sugar.

Evening Wrap-up

On the journey to wellness, we can find ourselves renewed—feeling like a new person. With that renewal comes opportunity to leave the cocoon of isolation that we set up for ourselves. When we leave our isolation, then we open the door to carry the burdens of others. Just as Ada became a new person and began helping others, so can we become new and find our own ways to engage the world.

Carry each other's burdens, and in this way you will fulfill the law of Christ. If anyone thinks they are something when they are not, they deceive themselves. Each one should test their own actions. Then they can take pride in themselves alone, without comparing themselves to someone else, for each one should carry their own load. . . . Therefore, as we have opportunity, let us do good to all people, especially to those who belong to the family of believers.

GALATIANS 6:2–5, 10

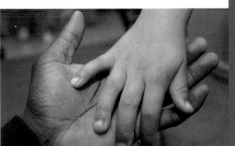

Renewing Spirit, help me to become a new person on this journey. Give me the strength to engage the world. Amen.

Morning Reflection

Renewal on the journey to wellness takes many different forms. One thing that we might notice, as we work toward managing our depression, is some lessening anxiety. As we learn to let go of control that we try to hold over everything, we can begin to feel like a new person. When we let go of control, other aspects of our personality can emerge. We can be more spontaneous and more joyous than if we are constantly trying to control everything around us.

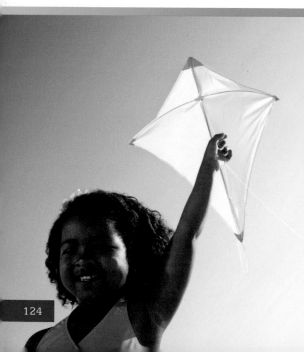

»Faith Life

Do you have a Bible verse that you feel "anchors" you? What is it? Today, take five minutes and write about that Bible verse in your journal. What has it meant to you in the past? Does it take on any new meaning on this journey?

»Medical

When was your last dental exam? If it has been more than six months, schedule an appointment today. A dentist can sometimes catch health problems that are otherwise "hidden," such as thyroid problems.

»Movement

Today, spend fifteen minutes doing abdominal-strength exercises. Standard sit-ups/crunches are a very good way to strengthen your core. Make sure that you do not strain your neck or back as you do those crunches!

> When we let go of control, other aspects of our personality can emerge.

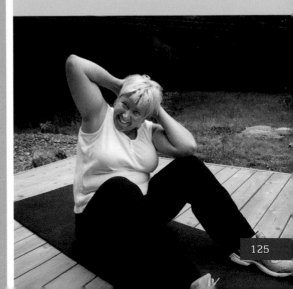

125

» Work

Do your coworkers know about your journey to wellness? Today, tell at least one of your coworkers about your journey. Often, workplaces can come together to strive toward wellness as a community. (Hint: If you are uncomfortable sharing that you are working to manage depression, just share your journey to overall wellness.)

» Emotional

Give yourself a rest today. Spend a half hour doing something you really enjoy. Read a book, listen to music, watch a television show, or take a bath. Just take care of yourself without worrying about the things that you "have to do" for thirty minutes.

» Family and Friends

Take a friend or family member and do something spontaneous today. Go to the park, a museum, or a movie. Let go of worrying about what you had planned for the day, and try to do something fun and spontaneous, even if you must stay home to do it.

» Nutrition

Some fats are necessary for balanced nutrition. Healthy fats can be found in avocados, seeds and nuts, olive oil, and fish. Today, prepare a meal using mostly healthy fats (no fried food or butter).

Evening Wrap-up

In some ways the journey to wellness is all about taking control of our lives: eating better, exercising regularly, engaging in self-care. But the journey to wellness is also about renewal and learning when to let go of the anxiety and stress that tends to control us (even when we think we are controlling it!). In Paul's letter to the Philippians, he admonishes them to let go of worry and instead trust that God will guard those things that we cannot control.

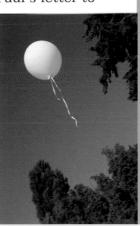

Rejoice in the Lord always. I will say it again: Rejoice! Let your gentleness be evident to all. The Lord is near. Do not be anxious about anything, but in every situation, by prayer and petition, with thanksgiving, present your requests to God. And the peace of God, which transcends all understanding, will guard your hearts and your minds in Christ Jesus.

PHILIPPIANS 4:4–7

Loving God, thank You for Your nearness and for listening to me when I call out. Help me to let go of worry and put my trust in You. Amen.

Morning Reflection

Sometimes when people talk about being renewed, they speak in the language of returning to the person they were born to be. This is particularly true in managing depression. While we are in the midst of our depression, it can be like standing outside of ourselves and watching while another person goes through the motions of our life. But on the journey to wellness, we can reunite with the person we know ourselves to be.

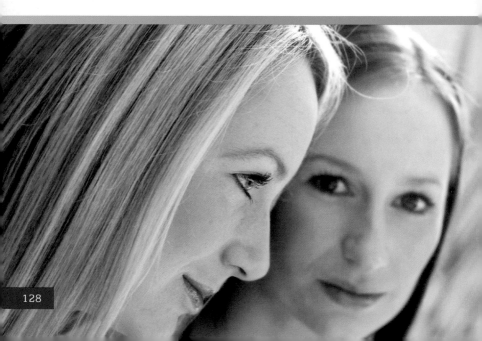

» Faith Life

Is there some part of your faith life that you used to enjoy and have stopped doing? Today think about a song, prayer, church group, or volunteer project that you enjoyed in the past. How can you re-involve yourself with that activity?

» Medical

Staying well-hydrated is very important to managing depression as well as to overall wellness. If you are not drinking at least eight eight-ounce glasses of water a day, then start drinking more water. (Hint: unsweetened, non-caffeinated tea or other caffeine- and sugar-free drinks count.)

» Movement

Swimming is excellent exercise. It is gentle on your joints and works just about every muscle group in your body. Today, if you have access to a pool, go for a swim—even spending ten minutes in the water will give you some great exercise. If you don't have access, see if there is a pool nearby.

» Work

Most workplaces have periods that are busy and periods that are slower. Whatever your work environment is like, find five minutes to breathe and stretch a little.

» Emotional

Have you had any experiences when you have felt "not yourself"? Today, take ten minutes and write in your journal about how you "came back" to yourself (if you did). If you have not experienced feeling this way, write about a time when you overcame a difficult emotional situation.

» Family and Friends

Sometimes your family and friends know "the real you" in a way that you have maybe lost sight of. Today, give an old friend a call and talk for a while. This can be a reminder of where your anchor is.

» Nutrition

Instead of drinking fruit juice, which has most of the healthy fiber juiced out of it, eat a whole piece of fruit. There is less sugar and just as much water in a piece of fruit.

Evening Wrap-up

Keep in mind that God knows us.

God knows our darkest moments along with our brightest, and God loves us through it all. When we are struggling with depression, we can feel the desire to hide the darkness from God and from others. But when we embrace the darkness within us and learn to deal with it, that is when our light can really shine through and we can be renewed in body and spirit.

You have searched me, LORD, and you know me. You know when I sit and when I rise; you perceive my thoughts from afar. You discern my going out and my lying down; you are familiar with all my ways. Before a word is on my tongue you, LORD, know it completely. You hem me in behind and before, and you lay your hand upon me.

PSALM 139:1–5

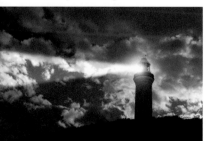

God of Light, You knit me together in my mother's womb. You know me. Help me to know myself as I continue on this journey. In Your holy name, Amen.

Morning Reflection

Though we will experience setbacks on the journey to wellness, it is important to keep in mind that the journey does change and renew us over time, sometimes without our even realizing it. It is at those times that we can look back and realize that something in us has been renewed—that we are somehow transformed and made different. And with the realization of that renewal, we can find relief. Today, we will turn our focus to the slow transformation and renewal that we experience over time.

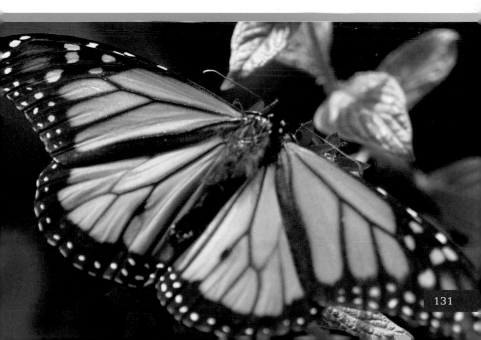

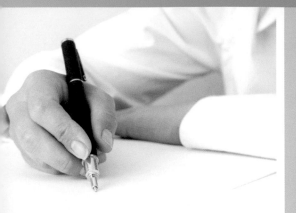

»Faith Life

Today, take five minutes and write ten words that describe your faith life. Then go back to Week One and compare your list now to your description then. Do you see how God has worked in your life?

»Medical

Over time, our over-the-counter medications will expire and be less effective. Today, clean out any old or expired medication, and make sure that you have a fully stocked first-aid kit at your home.

»Movement

Try incorporating movement into your small, everyday tasks. For example, do squats while you brush your teeth. Lunge your way from your bedroom to the kitchen. This can help you to incorporate movement into your day even when you don't have time to dedicate exclusively to exercising.

{ It is only natural that some of the sounds that we hear on a regular basis will change. }

»Work

Bring a stash of non-caffeinated, non-sweetened herbal teas into work. When you feel like drinking a cup of coffee, have a cup of herbal tea instead. That way you will be more hydrated, and you will avoid the bursts of energy and crashes that come with caffeine and sugar.

»Emotional

Many of us have had mountaintop experiences—moments when we feel everything clearly. But the real work is done in the valleys, when we can barely see the mountaintops. Today, write about times when you have been on the mountaintop and how those experiences translate to the work in the valleys.

»Family and Friends

Our personal relationships are instrumental in our transformations. Today, write in your journal about how your family and friends have influenced you on your journey to wellness.

»Nutrition

Go to the Internet to find healthy and interesting recipes. Try Church Health Reader at www.chreader.org, or other websites such as epicurious.com or mayoclinic.com, to search for healthy and seasonal recipes.

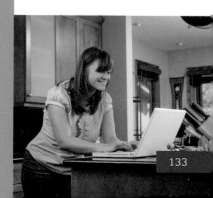

Evening Wrap-up

As he neared Damascus on his journey, suddenly a light from heaven flashed around him. He fell to the ground and heard a voice say to him, "Saul, Saul, why do you persecute me?" "Who are you, Lord?" Saul asked. "I am Jesus, whom you are persecuting," he replied. "Now get up and go into the city, and you will be told what you must do."

ACTS 9:3–6

We are all familiar with the story of how Saul became Paul on the road to Damascus. The conversion was quite literally marked by a light from heaven and Saul falling from his "high horse." But for most of us, the transformation is not quite so sudden and instant, nor do most of us change our names. That does not, however, mean that the transformation is any less meaningful or life changing. The changes that we make in our life and to our person are 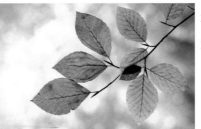 real and important.

Creator God, help me to notice the transformation in myself. In Your holy name, Amen.

Morning Reflection

Renewal and transformation not only take time, they take effort. The journey to wellness is about working toward a set of goals and constantly renewing the hope that we will get there, with time. As we continue on this journey, without actively seeking to renew our energy, we can burn out. The novelty wears off, life gets in the way, and we lose our momentum. So today, we will focus on the ways that we can renew our hope and energy for the journey.

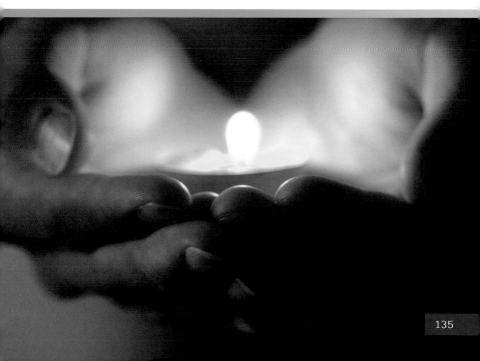

» Faith Life

What do you hope for in your faith life? What does hope mean? Take five minutes and write about hope as a part of your faith.

» Medical

Our bodies are designed so that when we exercise, our energy levels improve. Today, consider how energetic you feel as compared to when you started. How have you noticed a change in your body?

» Movement

Go for a walk today, walking as long as you can without exhausting yourself. Can you walk a good deal farther than you could before you started this journey? Imagine yourself in another six weeks and how far you will be able to walk then.

» Work

How has this journey impacted your work life thus far? Have you noticed changes in your attitude, your work ethic, your productivity? Consider how you have changed your work life today, and take note of your improvements.

» Emotional

Take an emotional inventory today. Write in your journal how you are feeling today and compare it to how you felt last week. Compare today's inventory to your inventory from Week One.

» Family and Friends

Often, our family and friends are not on exactly the same path as us. Today, if your family and friends do not seem to understand why you are on the journey, tell them your conversion story to help them to understand where you are coming from.

» Nutrition

If you eat canned fruit instead of fresh fruit, rinse the fruit off before you eat it. This will wash away some of the excess sugar and syrup that the fruit comes in.

Evening Wrap-up

As we continue on this journey,

our transformation may become more subtle and less exciting. But when the excitement dies down, and there is less to see on a day-to-day basis, the journey can lose its *oomph*. In the letter to the Hebrews, we are told, "Faith is being sure of what we hope for and certain of what we do not see." On our journey to wellness, we sometimes have to hope for what we cannot see.

Now faith is confidence in what we hope for and assurance about what we do not see. This is what the ancients were commended for. By faith we understand that the universe was formed at God's command, so that what is seen was not made out of what was visible.

Hebrews 11:1–3

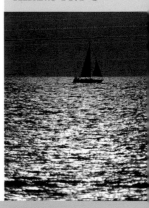

God who is Faithful, thank You for walking with me on this journey. Give me the faith and the hope to continue. In Your holy name, Amen.

Morning Reflection

As we work toward managing depression,
occasionally we need a cleansing. We need to clean out our bodies and spirits. When we take time to do that, we can find ourselves with a fresh start and a renewed sense of hope. When we are managing depression, that cleansing can sometimes mean "having a good cry" or finding a creative outlet for our emotions that we otherwise might keep bottled in. Those small things can really help us to have a fresh start.

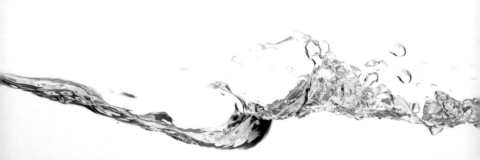

»Faith Life

There are many examples of washing and cleansing in the Bible. Today, think of a time of cleansing in your own life. Take five minutes to pray and write about that time.

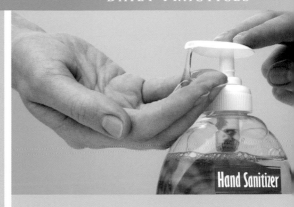

Hand Sanitizer

»Medical

One of the best ways to prevent both serious and minor illnesses (such as the common cold or staph infections) is to wash your hands frequently, particularly during times of the year when most people are inside. Also try keeping a bottle of alcohol-based hand-sanitizing gel with you.

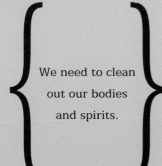

{ We need to clean out our bodies and spirits. }

»Movement

Swimming is an excellent form of exercise, but you don't have to worry about swimming laps. Lots of gyms offer aerobics classes in the water and can even teach you to swim! Today, think about whether a water aerobics class might be helpful and fun for you.

139

» Work

Today at work, if you are stuck sitting for long periods of time, try to move your feet by bouncing your legs up and down, or even rolling your ankles around. This will help maintain circulation in your legs and can help relieve pain or swelling that comes with that much sitting.

» Emotional

Have you had any major life changes recently? Depression is always more likely to strike around the time of a major change such as changing jobs or moving to a new city. Major life changes are major stressors, even when they are good changes. Give yourself plenty of room to process.

» Family and Friends

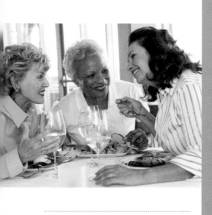

Today, go out to a favorite restaurant with some friends and/or family. Again, try to enjoy the company and the socializing more than the food. Enjoy the food, but make the social interaction the star of the evening.

» Nutrition

Vegetables can provide our body with a boost of energy. Today, try to incorporate an extra serving of vegetables in your day. Roasting some Brussels sprouts or steaming broccoli is a quick and easy way to add in an extra serving to your meal.

Evening Wrap-up

In the Christian tradition, we have an example of cleansing in baptism. We are washed clean with water and the Holy Spirit. Cleansing represents a new start—new beginnings. We discussed new beginnings in the first week of this journey. But the truth is, we can always use a good cleansing to begin again. The psalmist asks God for just this, and so can we—any time and any place. God will hear us and answer us.

Cleanse me with hyssop, and I will be clean; wash me, and I will be whiter than snow. Let me hear joy and gladness. . . . Create in me a pure heart, O God, and renew a steadfast spirit within me. Do not cast me from your presence or take your Holy Spirit from me. Restore to me the joy of your salvation and grant me a willing spirit, to sustain me.

PSALM 51:7–8, 10–12

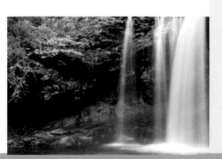

Refreshing Spirit, thank You for Your constant promise of renewal and new beginnings. Give me the courage to begin again whenever I need it. Amen.

Morning Reflection

Congratulations! We have arrived at the end of the fifth week. At this point in our journey, we can look back at all that we have done and be very pleased with our work. Furthermore, as we continue to work on managing depression, we can look back into darkness and hopefully begin to look forward into light. As we travel on from here, we will work to embrace the light that lies ahead of us.

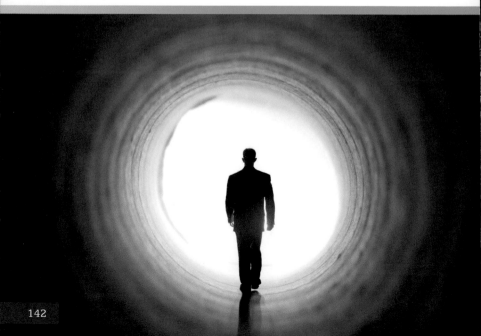

»Faith Life

Talk to your pastor or another leader in your faith community about your journey. This person could be a very valuable resource as you continue the journey to wellness and managing depression.

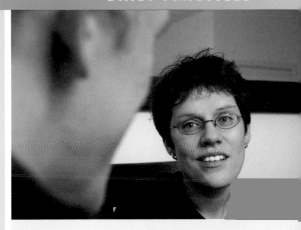

»Medical

Are you maintaining a good sleep routine? If you are having difficulty sleeping, even after taking steps to improve your sleep, talk to your doctor. Sleep disorders do exist, and many are easily treatable.

»Movement

You can use everyday items in your home to get a good workout—you do not need to go to the gym. Try doing bicep curls with bottles of water, or wall push-ups. Be creative with your exercise!

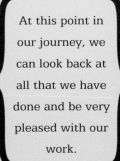

At this point in our journey, we can look back at all that we have done and be very pleased with our work.

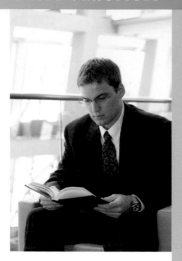

»Work

Bring a good book with you to work. When you have breaks, or if you have lunch by yourself, take a few minutes and read. Reading a good book can give you a chance to "escape," even if it is only for a few minutes.

»Emotional

Today, try to find a time and place to watch a beautiful sunrise or sunset. If it happens to be cloudy, make plans to do so in a few days. Witnessing the light of the sun can be an emotionally uplifting experience.

»Family and Friends

A large part of any healing is our support system. Today, have a conversation with the members of your family and friends who are an important part of your support system. Tell them what healing on this journey looks like for you.

»Nutrition

Try cooking a "meatless" meal today. Use beans, nuts, and/or tofu to add some protein to vegetables and whole grains for a nutritious, low-fat dinner.

Evening Wrap-up

We have completed five weeks:

thirty-five days. Soon, this part of the journey will be done, and we will continue the journey to wellness in other ways. But however we continue, we can be assured that God walks with us and gives us light. God offers us light and hope even when we are in darkness. On the journey to wellness, we can depend on that light from this point forward.

"Arise, shine, for your light has come, and the glory of the Lord rises upon you. See, darkness covers the earth and thick darkness is over the peoples, but the Lord rises upon you and his glory appears over you. . . . The sun will no more be your light by day, nor will the brightness of the moon shine on you, for the Lord will be your everlasting light, and your God will be your glory."

Isaiah 60:1–2, 19

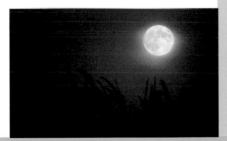

Loving God, thank You for walking this journey with me and giving me the strength to make it this far. Continue to walk with me, I pray, Amen.

Dawn does not remember feeling depressed.

She just remembers, as a child, wondering why everyone else seemed so happy all the time. "I remember looking at my parents and thinking there was something wrong with them." But over time, she started to believe that there was something wrong with *her*. When she became a teenager, she had a great deal of difficulty sustaining friendships, and high school was extraordinarily difficult. "I had this theory that I was a mistake. I didn't fit in this world."

When Dawn was eighteen years old, she skipped school and made her first suicide attempt. She would attempt suicide one more time before she really got the help she needed. "In the course of treatment, I found a psychiatrist who finally seemed to understand that I didn't know how to describe what was wrong because I'd never felt another way!" Dawn was diagnosed with severe clinical depression and was prescribed antidepressants.

With the antidepressants stabilizing her mood, Dawn began attending a church. She found something there that she had never felt in her whole life—belonging. "For the first time, I felt like I had a place in the world. I was beginning to heal."

Dawn came to the Church Health Center about six years ago with some of her friends from church. She now exercises regularly, eats a balanced diet, and finds that most of the time she is content. She now says that, "The greatest gift that God has given me is a place where I belong."

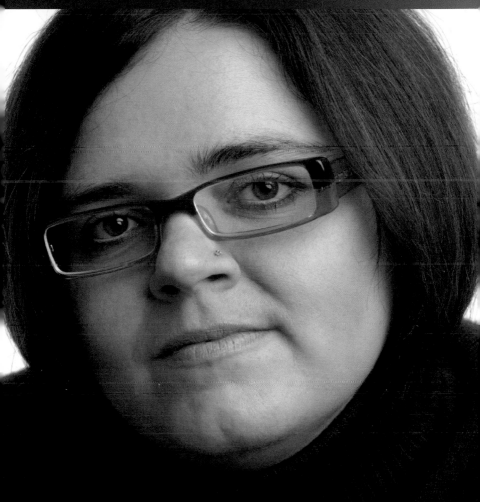

"For the first time, I felt like I had a place in the world. I was beginning to heal."

Morning Reflection

Some of us began this journey with a stark wake-up call that something had to change. Others of us perhaps just had a nagging feeling that we wanted to feel better. However we started, we have now arrived at the sixth week—the end of this journey—and we each have an individual and unique story that we can start to tell. Today we will turn our focus to what each of our stories means.

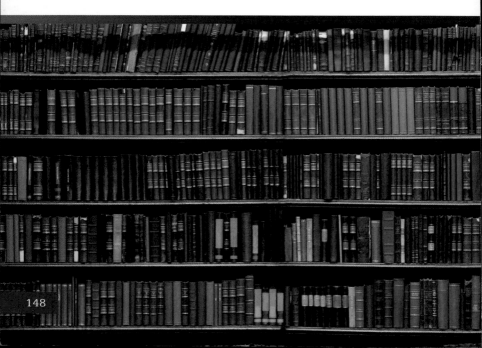

»Faith Life

Today, try a walking meditation. Go for a slow walk around your neighborhood (or even your backyard). Try to quiet your mind and just feel yourself moving.

»Medical

At this point in the journey, it may be time to start increasing your exercise level.
If you are going to engage in any kind of rigorous exercise program, talk to your doctor before you start. He or she can help you start a program safely.

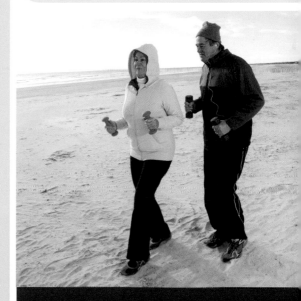

{
We each have an individual and unique story that we can start to tell.
}

»Movement

Go for a walk today and pick up the pace.
Swing your arms, and get your heart rate up. If you feel up for it, try walking with some small (two-to-five-pound) hand weights.

149

»Work

If you have stairs at work, take the stairs instead of the elevator. You will burn more calories getting to work, and you will save energy from using the elevators.

»Emotional

An important part of the journey from here can be learning how to tell your story. Today, take ten minutes, think back, and write about the beginning of your journey. It could be the day you picked up this book or the day you decided you needed a change.

»Family and Friends

Remember that family dinners are a great way to share your experiences of the day and to try out new recipes. Today, try to share a little bit of your story with your family as you share a meal.

»Nutrition

Make a standard list for the grocery store using the nutritional lessons that you have learned over the course of the last six weeks. You can use this list as a template for your grocery lists each week.

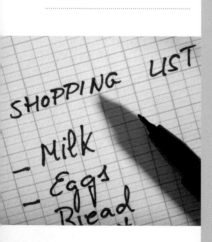

Evening Wrap-up

All of us have a story of the beginning of our journey. We can see where we came from, and we can remember the moment when we "woke from our slumber." As we move forward on our journey, it will be important to remember where our stories begin. Because if we remember where our story begins, then we can see God's hand in our journey when we look back at our story. We can look back and see God's hand and be thankful that we are now awake.

And do this, understanding the present time: The hour has already come for you to wake up from your slumber, because our salvation is nearer now than when we first believed. The night is nearly over; the day is almost here. So let us put aside the deeds of darkness and put on the armor of light.

ROMANS 13:11–12

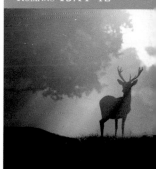

God of the beginning, the middle, and the end, thank You for walking this journey with me. Help me to remember my story as I continue on this journey to wellness. In Your holy name, Amen.

Morning Reflection

On this journey to wellness, we are coming, bit by bit, to know ourselves in ways that we had not known ourselves before. We have stretched our limits and learned new boundaries. The knowledge that we are gaining of ourselves will be very important as we move into the journey beyond these six weeks. The self-knowledge and self-awareness gained on this journey are particularly critical for managing depression. So today, we will focus not just on self-awareness but also on learning to see ourselves through God's eyes.

»Faith Life

We have all heard the commandment to "love your neighbor as yourself." But the first step in "love your neighbor as yourself" is to love yourself. Today, remember that God loves you, and spend five minutes writing about what it means to love yourself.

{
We have stretched our limits and learned new boundaries.
}

»Medical

Trust that you know your body and how it works. If something feels "off" to you, talk to your doctor, even if you don't know exactly what you are describing. Your doctor can ask questions to help you articulate what is wrong.

»Movement

Over the course of the last six weeks, you have come to know your body and how your body moves. Today, spend some time exercising in your favorite way. Go for a walk, do some jumping jacks, try yoga. Let your body move the way you want it to.

153

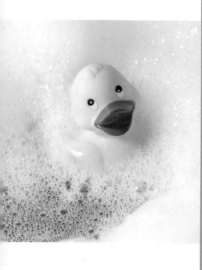

» Work

At work, try gathering some of your colleagues for wellness activities. Organize a bike-riding group to take a ride after hours or a lunch-break walking group. This will help you to build a community in your workplace and will help motivate you to continue wellness at work.

» Emotional

Today, take a hot bath to relax. Breathe in the steam, let your muscles go soft, close your eyes, and enjoy the quiet. If you feel comfortable, put on some music and/or light a candle to let yourself relax even more.

» Family and Friends

When you plan activities with your friends and family, make plans that do not necessarily revolve around food. Go to the park or a museum. This will help you to make family outings more active.

» Nutrition

For a quick, easy, and healthy meal, sauté some vegetables in olive oil and serve over brown rice. Add some beans and nuts for added protein, and be sure to season with some herbs, such as basil or marjoram.

Evening Wrap-up

On this journey, we are learning how to know ourselves. But even as we are working to know ourselves, we can rest assured that God knows us, inside and out. God knit us together, from a time even before we were born. Imagine being so known and cared for! God loves us and cares for our every fiber. And as we move forward on the journey, we can learn to know and love ourselves, too.

For you created my inmost being; you knit me together in my mother's womb. I praise you because I am fearfully and wonderfully made; your works are wonderful, I know that full well. My frame was not hidden from you when I was made in the secret place, when I was woven together in the depths of the earth. Your eyes saw my unformed body; all the days ordained for me were written in your book before one of them came to be.

Psalm 139:13–16

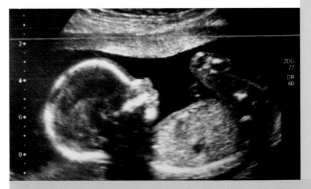

Loving God, I know that I am fearfully and wonderfully made. Help me always to know the care that You have shown me. In Your holy name, Amen.

Morning Reflection

As we approach the end of our six-week journey, we must remember that the journey does not stop with the end of this book. Managing depression and the overall journey toward wellness are lifelong journeys. And so, as we approach the end of this leg of the journey, we must prepare for the next steps that we'll take. After all, wellness is not a goal that can be attained and then left behind. So today we will begin planning for those next steps.

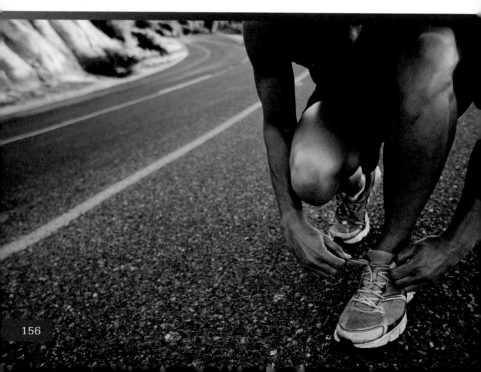

» Faith Life

As we continue on the journey, it is important to find anchor points. Today, spend five minutes writing about the anchor points in your life. What gives you hope as you continue on the journey?

» Medical

Practicing good preventive medicine is crucial for wellness. Have a conversation with your doctor about any screenings and tests that you might need to have.

» Movement

If you run to the store to buy a gallon of milk, carry the milk with you instead of putting it in your cart. Then, while you stand in line, do some alternating bicep curls with it.

» Work

Bring an insulated lunch bag to work with some raw chopped vegetables such as celery, carrots, and red bell peppers to snack on when you get hungry. If you want to add a little spice, throw in a few radishes as well.

» Emotional

Branching out into the next part of the journey can be intimidating. Today, make a list of the activities that you have discovered that work to help you manage your stress.

» Family and Friends

Your family and friends will be very important to your journey. Today, try to set up a regular walking time with (at least) one of your friends or family members. Having a regular time will help you to get into (and continue in) the habit of walking.

» Nutrition

Now that you have introduced some new foods into your diet, think about taking your cooking skills to the next level. Find a healthy cooking class or look for a new book or website with recipes. Try to develop a new favorite dish that you can prepare on your own.

Praise be to the God and Father of our Lord Jesus Christ! In his great mercy he has given us new birth into a living hope through the resurrection of Jesus Christ from the dead, and into an inheritance that can never perish, spoil or fade. This inheritance is kept in heaven for you, who through faith are shielded by God's power until the coming of the salvation that is ready to be revealed in the last time.

1 PETER 1:3–5

Evening Wrap-up

This journey to wellness is about new birth and fresh starts. We have gained skills and knowledge that will help us to be healthy and manage our depression. And so at this point, we need never to cease hoping that our lives can change. Peter reminds us that God's hope is always the hope for new life through the resurrection of Jesus Christ.

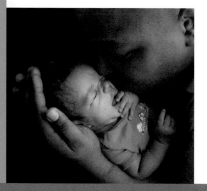

Giving God, help me today as I plan my next steps. Grant me hope and encouragement for the journey ahead. In Your holy name, Amen.

Morning Reflection

As we approach the final stretch of our six-week journey, we need to be reminded that we are not alone on the journey. Though it is true that we are, in most cases, trying to change individual habits, the people who surround us can give us encouragement. Furthermore, encouraging others on the wellness journey can help us to feel encouraged ourselves. Reaching out to others is particularly important as we learn to manage our depression.

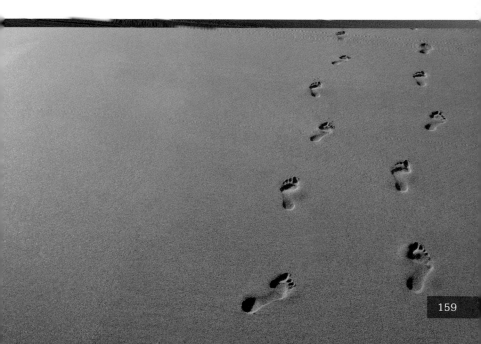

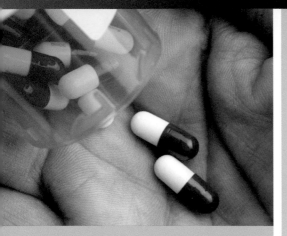

»Faith Life

**Does your faith commu-
nity have Sunday school
programs?** Today, consider
starting up a Sunday school
program that is centered
on the wellness journey.
Encourage other members
of your faith community to
live wellness-oriented lives.

»Medical

**Remember that medication is not a
magical pill.** When your physician writes a
prescription for a medication, ask questions
about what lifestyle changes you should
be making along with the medication to be
healthier.

»Movement

**Today, before you eat dinner, do some
cardio exercises.** Go for a walk, jog in place
for five minutes, or do thirty jumping jacks.
Exercising before eating will make you feel
healthier, and will in turn motivate you to eat
healthier.

> We need to be
> reminded that we
> are not alone on
> the journey.

»Work

If there is someone at your work who shares your particular lunchtime, and perhaps is interested in eating healthy meals, adopt that person as a lunch buddy. Take turns bringing in new, healthy dishes to try.

»Emotional

When we feel alone, we can become despondent, and it can really halt our progress in managing depression. Today, spend five minutes writing about the many ways in which you are not alone.

»Family and Friends

Your family and friends can be of great support, but it can also be good to seek support from people who are going through a very similar experience as you. Support groups exist at gyms and wellness centers as well as online. Find a group that you can belong to.

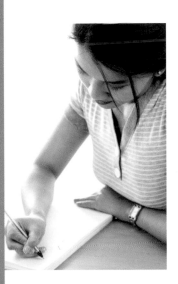

»Nutrition

An important piece of eating well is eating together. Today, make a menu of what you would like to serve at a dinner with friends and make plans for the dinner. It may be tomorrow or weeks ahead, but make plans now so you can enjoy eating with others.

161

"My command is this: Love each other as I have loved you. Greater love has no one than this: to lay down one's life for one's friends. You are my friends if you do what I command. . . . I chose you and appointed you so that you might go and bear fruit— fruit that will last. . . . This is my command: Love each other."

JOHN 15:12–14, 16–17

Evening Wrap-up

As you continue on this journey,

keep in mind that you are loved deeply by Jesus Christ, who laid down His life so that we might live. But as we bask in the light of Christ's love, we are also called to one another. We are called to live in community, to support one another, and to "bear fruit. . .that will last." Loving ourselves and each other is fruit that will last.

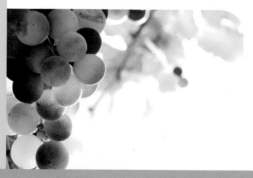

Life-sustaining Lord, thank You for loving me. Give me the strength to continue on this journey and to encourage others who are also on the journey. In Your holy name, Amen.

Morning Reflection

Today is Day 40—congratulations! You have made it forty days! Over the past six weeks you have gained the skills necessary to continue on your journey toward wellness. Setbacks will probably happen from time to time, but in the last six weeks, you have set up a foundation that you can return to when needed. Managing our depression is about knowing that, whatever unexpected turns the journey brings, we can live a full and abundant life.

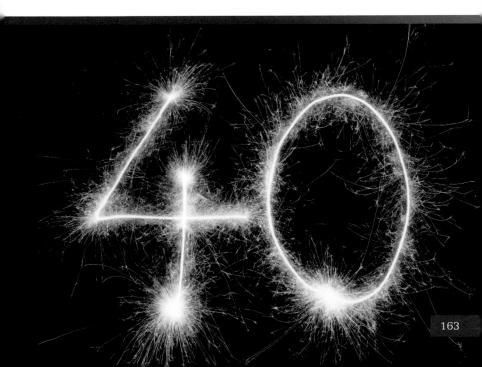

» Faith Life

What does this milestone mean for you? Today, think about how your faith has changed along this journey. Did you believe you would get here? How has God sustained you through this journey? How would you like to carry this experience forward?

» Medical

Don't wait to go to a doctor until you are sick. If you change health care providers, try to get to know them while you are healthy. It is much easier for doctors to treat you when they know what the "healthy you" is like.

» Movement

In celebration of life in abundance, put on some music and dance today. Bounce around, get your heart rate up, and don't forget to use your arms!

» Work

If you need to go out to lunch for work, ask for a "to go" box to come out with your food. If the portions are larger than what is healthy (as is the case at most restaurants), put half of your order in the box before you eat.

» Emotional

Today, take your last emotional inventory of this journey. As you write, reflect on the last six weeks, and consider how you are feeling in light of the journey to this point.

» Family and Friends

Today, prepare a meal for your friends and family that you have never prepared before. Get your guests to help you prepare the meal, chopping vegetables or stirring the pot as things cook.

» Nutrition

Do not skip breakfast! If you want a change from the usual cereal, try eating leftovers from last night's dinner for breakfast. That'll get you at least a serving of vegetables to start out the day.

Evening Wrap-up

Remember that God gives us abundant grace through Jesus Christ and that we are not only given abundant grace in spirit, but in our whole selves and our whole lives. This journey to wellness is about responding appropriately to that abundant grace that Jesus Christ grants us. When we care for ourselves, we are caring for God's creation—the very thing that Jesus came to save.

For if, by the trespass of the one man, death reigned through that one man, how much more will those who receive God's abundant provision of grace and of the gift of righteousness reign in life through the one man, Jesus Christ!

ROMANS 5:17

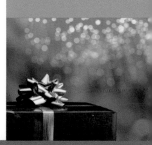

God of the journey, thank You for walking with me on this journey, and for the abundant grace that You give me. Help me today and all days to live my life to abundance in wellness and in grace. In Your holy name, Amen.

Morning Reflection

Now that the forty days are over, today will be a day of review. When we started out this journey, we had to assess where we were in order to set goals for the journey. In a similar manner, we have to assess where we are again, so that we can know where we need to go from here. We need to see our successes as well as our setbacks, so that we know where we still need to work.

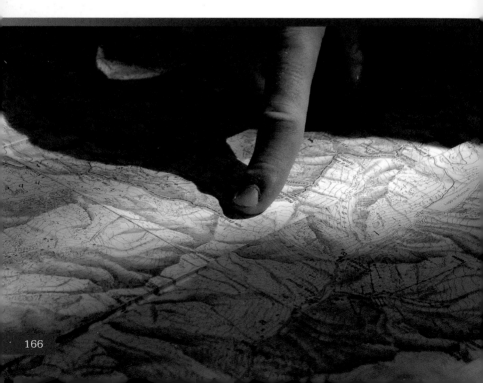

»Faith Life

When we started, you wrote a short description, and later ten words, describing your faith life. Again, take five minutes and write ten words describing your faith life now. Then compare the two lists. What has changed? What has stayed the same?

»Medical

What are your medical concerns now? Are they significantly different from what they were six weeks ago? Write down your current medical concerns, but do not get rid of your old list of concerns.

»Movement

Go for a walk today, and walk as far as you can go. How far could you walk the first time you did this? Can you feel the improvement in the way your body is reacting to the walking?

> We need to see our successes as well as our setbacks, so that we know where we still need to work.

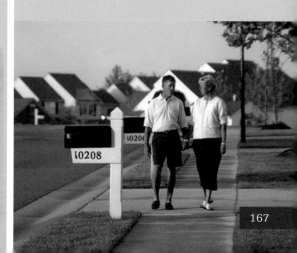

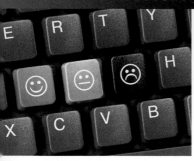

» Work

What has changed about your work environment? Are you drinking more water? Are you eating healthier snacks? Are you getting a little exercise throughout the day?

» Emotional

What has changed in your emotional wellness? Have you found ways to change your emotional patterns? Do you feel different now than you did when you started?

» Family and Friends

What have your family and friends thought about your journey? Can they see a difference in you? Take a moment today and ask one or two of them.

» Nutrition

What are the foods that you like to eat now, after the six weeks are over? Have any new healthy foods made it onto the list?

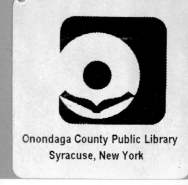

Evening Wrap-up

The last six weeks have been challenging in a variety of ways. You have been asked to try vastly new things, from food to exercises. You have been asked to step outside of your comfort zone, explore emotions that most of us do not take the time to explore regularly. But the journey—at least this part of the journey—is finished. And you have finished the race. For that, you ought to be very proud and thankful. You have run the race, and God has been running right beside you. Remember as you continue from this point, God runs the race with you. God gives us all strength and endurance when we most need it, and God cheers when we cross the finish line.

I have fought the good fight, I have finished the race, I have kept the faith.

2 TIMOTHY 4:7

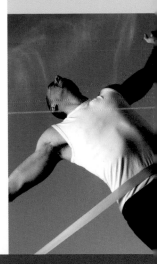

Merciful God, thank You for the gift of wellness. Help me to continue on this journey with endurance and bravery. In Your holy name, Amen.

Morning Reflection

With the six weeks completed, it can certainly feel like the journey is over. However, as we have said before, the journey has really only just begun. The journey to wellness and to managing depression is never over. Life will offer us many surprises along the way, and it will be part of the journey to adapt as life happens. Today, as we close this chapter on the journey, we look ahead to continue the lessons learned on this journey.

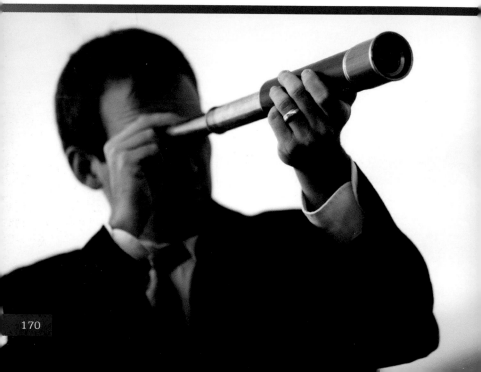

»Faith Life

As you continue on this journey, remember to take time to pray or meditate each day. Prayer and meditation can keep you connected to your purpose and your anchor.

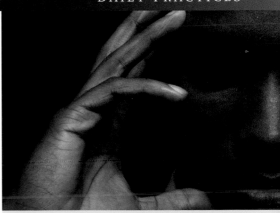

»Medical

Take all medication exactly as prescribed, and do not be afraid to talk to your doctor about anything. The best way to stay medically healthy is to have open communication with your physician.

{ The journey to wellness is never over. }

»Movement

Move everywhere. Find ways to add a few steps to your day in everything that you do. A great goal would be to add two hundred steps to each day, which will help your body to burn calories more efficiently each day.

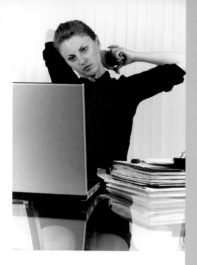

»Work

Try to find time in your day to exercise even a little bit. It will help break up the monotony of the day and will help you to add a few steps. Also, avoid office junk food. Instead, opt for healthy snacks and lunches.

»Emotional

To continue to manage your depression, if you are not already seeing a counselor, try going to one. Ask your pastor or doctor for a recommendation.

»Family and Friends

Remember that your family and friends are your support system. When you are struggling, do not be afraid to lean on them for support, and when you have succeeded, do not be afraid to celebrate with them.

»Nutrition

Make your calories count. Enjoy all of the wonderful colors and flavors of God's creation as you prepare meals using whole grains, a variety of fruits and vegetables, and lean meats—but do let yourself splurge on occasion!

Evening Wrap-up

It has been a long journey to this point, but you have been given many tools to continue the journey. You will find other tools to add to your toolbox, and you will have setbacks. But remember that God walks with you, and God can grant you peace, even when you have a difficult time finding it for yourself.

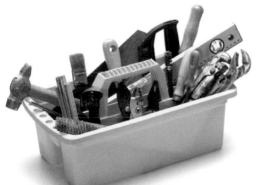

Finally, brothers and sisters, whatever is true, whatever is noble, whatever is right, whatever is pure, whatever is lovely, whatever is admirable—if anything is excellent or praiseworthy—think about such things. Whatever you have learned or received or heard from me, or seen in me—put it into practice. And the God of peace will be with you.

PHILIPPIANS 4:8–9

Lord of the future, be with me as I continue on this journey. Help me to remember the things I have learned, and help me to continue learning. I will continue to strive to honor my body and my whole self, Your creation. In Your holy name, Amen.

Recommended Reading and Resources:

Book
The Depression Workbook by Mary Ellen Copeland (available through www.mentalhealthrecovery.com)

Websites
The Church Health Reader: www.chreader.org

The National Alliance on Mental Illness: http://NAMI.org

The Depression and Bipolar Support Alliance: http://www.dbsalliance.org

The National Depression Screening Site: http://mentalhealthscreening.org/events/national depreccion-screening-day.aspx

WebMD Depression Information: http://www.webmd.com/depression/default.htm

Action Plan for Prevention and Recovery: http://store.samhsa.gov/product/SMA-3720

40 DAYS TO BETTER LIVING

A series of practical books dealing with specific health issues

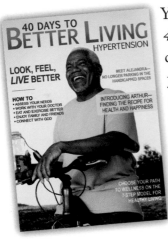

You want to feel better—and *40 Days to Better Living* provides clear, manageable steps to get you there through life-changing attitudes and actions. If you're ready to live better, select one or more elements of the Seven-Step Model for Healthy Living—Faith Life, Medical, Movement, Work, Emotional, Family and Friends, and Nutrition—and follow the forty-day plan to improve your life, just a bit, day by day. With plenty of practical advice, biblical encouragement, and stories of real people who have taken the same journey, this may be the most important book you read this year!

Bimonthly release schedule.

Titles to include:

Optimal Health / Hypertension / Depression / Rest and Relaxation / Weight Management / Stress Management / Aging / Addiction / Diabetes / Anxiety / Caregiving

Available wherever Christian books are sold.